FOOD SCIENCE AND TECHNOLOGY

NUTRACEUTICALS

PROSPECTS, SOURCES AND ROLE IN HEALTH AND DISEASE

FOOD SCIENCE AND TECHNOLOGY

Additional books in this series can be found on Nova's website under the Series tab.

Additional e-books in this series can be found on Nova's website under the eBooks tab.

FOOD SCIENCE AND TECHNOLOGY

NUTRACEUTICALS

PROSPECTS, SOURCES AND ROLE IN HEALTH AND DISEASE

NOBORU MOTOHASHI
EDITOR

nova
biomedical
New York

Library of Congress Cataloging-in-Publication Data

ISBN: 978-1-53611-785-1

Library of Congress Control Number: 2017937345

Published by Nova Science Publishers, Inc. † New York

CONTENTS

PREFACE

Bioactive phytochemicals contribute immensely to the operations and functions that occur within human beings. Scientists have coined the term "nutraceuticals" to describe any plant-based biochemical substances that positively affect physical condition and status. They promote health benefits and serve many purposes, such as acting as antioxidants, cancer inhibitors, hepatoprotectants, hypertensive inhibitors, and possessing antidiabetic and antidepressant properties, among other qualities. With these characteristics in mind, the authors describe how these nutraceuticals aid in the prevention and treatments of diseases. The authors intend for their research to aid in the further exploration and discovery of new drug designs and applications for nutraceuticals.

Chapter 1 – The common definition of nutraceuticals is based on the literature. Many kinds of psychotropic drugs (minor tranquilizers) and antipsychotic drugs (major tranquilizers) have been used in treatments of mental illness such as depression and schizophrenia. The main two drugs generally come with adverse effects. Combined administration of conventional psychotropic medicines or antipsychotic drugs with plant-derived components has been tried for the increased drug effect. Combined administration may be especially beneficial for treatment of depression and schizophrenia as a complementary and alternative medicine (CAM). Omega-3 fatty acids such as docosapentaenoic acid (DPA), docosahexaenoic acid (DHA), linoleic acid (LA), and arachidonic acid (AA) showed an improved effect for schizophrenia. A sugar alcohol inositol, a six-fold alcohol (polyol) of cyclohexane, showed improved effect for panic disorder and depression, and combined administration of inositol with selective serotonin reuptake inhibitors (SSRI) enhanced the antidepressant effect. Folic acid (folate) and folinic acid (leucovorin) are involved in folate deficiency during early neurodevelopment predisposed to schizophrenia. *S*-adenosylmethionine (SAMe) of naturally occurring food plant components showed from clinical meta-analysis a significant effect for treatment of depression. This chapter reviews the definition of nutraceuticals and the enhancement effect by combined administration of conventional psychotropic medicines or antipsychotic drugs with plant-derived components such as omega-3 fatty acids (ω-3 FAc), inositol (*myo*-inositol), folate and leucovorin, and SAMe for improvement and treament of depression and schizophrenia.

Chapter 2 – Beans have been consumed since prehispanic times and, nowadays, are one of the most eaten legumes worldwide. Among ~70 varieties, beans are now considered as functional foods due to the presence of different phytochemicals, e.g., phenolic compounds. These have been reported to exhibit a wide variety of nutraceutic effects, including those oriented to weight-control and therefore, obesity. Although evidence of both observational and experimental studies has revealed positive tendencies related to bean consumption/ supplementation and weight-loss, more rigorous trials are needed in order to consider this functional food within the every-day therapeutics of obesity.

Chapter 3 – Rice bran is the most abundant by-product obtained from the rice (*Oryza sativa*) milling process. The whole rice grain is rich in bioactive compounds which are found mainly in the bran. This bran contains naturally-occurring antioxidants, mainly γ-oryzanol, tocopherols, tocotrienols and polyphenols. Moreover, proteins from rice bran have a high nutritional value. Despite having components of biological significance, the nutritional use of rice bran is limited due to its poor water-solubility and to the lipid deterioration that starts soon after bran removal. Using enzymatic technology, the authors group has developed a process that enables a stable, water-soluble enzymatic extract (RBEE) to be obtained from rice bran. The enzymatic process increases the concentration of minor functional components, making RBEE rich in bioactive compounds. Thus, RBEE has antioxidant and hypocholesterolemic properties, as well as antiproliferative and inmuno-activatory abilities. Interestingly, in animal models an RBEE-supplemented diet showed beneficial effects on the cardiovascular system. RBEE ameliorates cardio-metabolic risk factors in obese Zucker rats, as well as ameliorating the proinflamatory response and microvascular alterations associated with obesity. Moreover, RBEE also prevents high-fat diet-induced inflammation in adipose tissue of C57BL/6J mice, as well as preventing vascular impairment in ApoE−/− mice.

Chapter 4 – The main objective of this chapter is to provide information on a substance that has revolutionized studies in various scientific fields and is expected to have a great impact on the study of natural substances with nutraceutical properties. Phyto-melatonin (plant melatonin) is chemically related to amino acids but with very diverse properties. The interest in phyto-melatonin is due to its outstanding action at cellular and physiological level, while its plant origin offers many opportunities because it is a natural compound. An overview on its origin, its action in plants in general and in particular plant species with high levels of phyto-melatonin, and its use as a nutraceutical, is present. The beneficial effects that it may have on human health are also analyzed. The differences between synthetic melatonin and phyto-melatonin, according to their origin and purity, will be presented. Finally, a brief discussion on the current market for phyto-melatonin and its limits and possibilities is presented.

In: Nutraceuticals
Editor: Noboru Motohashi

ISBN: 978-1-53611-785-1

Chapter 1

NUTRACEUTICALS AS COMPLEMENTARY AND ALTERNATIVE MEDICINE: THE ADJUVANT EFFECT WITH DEPRESSION AND SCHIZOPHRENIA

Noboru Motohashi*

Meiji Pharmaceutical University, Noshio, Kiyose-shi, Tokyo, Japan

ABSTRACT

The common definition of nutraceuticals is based on the literature. Many kinds of psychotropic drugs (minor tranquilizers) and antipsychotic drugs (major tranquilizers) have been used in treatments of mental illness such as depression and schizophrenia. The main two drugs generally come with adverse effects. Combined administration of conventional psychotropic medicines or antipsychotic drugs with plant-derived components has been tried for the increased drug effect. Combined administration may be especially beneficial for treatment of depression and schizophrenia as a complementary and alternative medicine (CAM).

Omega-3 fatty acids such as docosapentaenoic acid (DPA), docosahexaenoic acid (DHA), linoleic acid (LA), and arachidonic acid (AA) showed an improved effect for schizophrenia. A sugar alcohol inositol, a six-fold alcohol (polyol) of cyclohexane, showed improved

* Corresponding author email: noborumotohashi@jcom.home.ne.jp.

effect for panic disorder and depression, and combined administration of inositol with selective serotonin reuptake inhibitors (SSRI) enhanced the antidepressant effect. Folic acid (folate) and folinic acid (leucovorin) are involved in folate deficiency during early neurodevelopment predisposed to schizophrenia. *S*-adenosylmethionine (SAMe) of naturally occurring food plant components showed from clinical meta-analysis a significant effect for treatment of depression.

This chapter reviews the definition of nutraceuticals and the enhancement effect by combined administration of conventional psychotropic medicines or antipsychotic drugs with plant-derived components such as omega-3 fatty acids (ω-3 FAc), inositol (*myo*-inositol), folate and leucovorin, and SAMe for improvement and treament of depression and schizophrenia.

Keywords: nutraceuticals, depression, schizophrenias, selective serotonin reuptake inhibitors (SSRIs), antidepressants, *S*-adenosyl-L-methionine (SAMe), intention-to-treat (ITT) analysis

ABBREVIATIONS

docosahexaenoic acid (DHA. 22:6n3. C22:6(ω-3). 22:6n3. 1)
eicosapentaenoic acid (EPA. C20:5(ω–3). 20:5n3. 2)
α-linolenic acid (linolenic acid. ALA. 18:3(n-3), 18:3($\Delta^{9,12,15}$), 18:3n3. 3)
ethyl eicosapentaenoic acid (E-EPA. 4)
arachidonic acid (AA. C20:4(ω-6). 20:4n6. 5)
linoleic acid (LA, 18:2n6(ω-6). 6)
5-hydroxyindoleacetic acid (5-HIAA. 7)
serotonin (5HT, 5-hydroxytryptamine. 8)
docosapentaenoic acid (DPA. 22:5n3. C22:5(ω-3). 9)
homovanillic acid (HVA. 10)
vitamin E (11)
citalopram (12)
fluoxetine (13)
fluvoxamine (14)
mirtazapine (15)
moclobemide (16)
paroxetine (17)
trazodone (18)
inositol (*myo*-inositol. MI. vitamin B8. 19)

phytic acid (*myo*-inositol-1,2,3,4,5,6-hexaphosphate. *cis*-1,2,3,5-*trans*-4,6-cyclohexanehexol. 20)
glucose (21)
chlorpromazine (CPZ. 22)
scyllo-inositol (23)
N-acetylaspartate (NAA. 24)
taurine (25)
methylfolate (levomefolic acid. 26)
folinic acid (leucovorin. 27)
folic acid (folate. 28)
homocysteine (29)
vitamin B12 (30)
S-adenosyl-L-methionine (SAMe. 31)
cystathionine (32)
cysteine (33)
glutathione (GSH. gamma-L-Glu-L-Cys-Gly. 34)
decarboxylated SAMe (deca-SAMe. decarboxylated *S*-adenosylmethionine. 35)
methyl-thioadenosine (MTA. 36)
methionine (37)
S-adenosyl-L-methionine tosylate (SAMe-tosylate. 38)
venlafaxine (39)
escitalopram (40)
sertraline (41)
Aβ: amyloid-β
Abeta40: amyloid beta40 peptide
Abeta42: amyloid beta42 peptide
AD: Alzheimer's disease
ADD: attention deficit disorder
ADHD: attention deficit hyperactivity disorder
AIDS virus: acquired immune deficiency syndrome virus
aMCI: amnestic mild cognitive impairment
APPswe: amyloid precursor protein swe
Brown Goodwin Score: Brown Goodwin Lifetime History of Aggression Scale
Buss Durkee Score: Buss Durkee Hostility Inventory
CAM: complementary and alternative medicine
CDRS: Calgary depression rating scale
CI: cumulative incidence

CNS: central nervous system
CNVs: copy-number variants
COPD: chronic obstructive pulmonary disease
CRoPS: complexity reduction of polymorphic sequences
CSF: cerebrospinal fluid
DALYs: disability-adjusted life years
DSM-IV: *Diagnostic and Statistical Manual of Mental Disorders, 4th ed.*
ECT: electroconvulsive therapy
EX1 cohort: exposed birth cohorts of August 1 through October 14, 1945
EX2 cohort: exposed birth cohorts of October 15 through December 31, 1945
ω-3FAc: omega-3 fatty acids
fibrillar Aβ: fibrillar amyloid-β
FLD: frontal lobe dementia
HAM-D17: 17-item Hamilton depression scale
HDSS: Hamilton depression scale score
1H-MRS: proton magnetic resonance spectroscopy
HIV: human immunodeficiency virus
HR-MAS: high resolution magic angle spinning
HRSD: Hamilton rating scale for depression
$HRSD_{21}$: 21-item version of the Hamilton rating scale for depression
ω-3HUFAs: omega-3 highly unsaturated fatty acids
IHD: ischaemic heart disease
ITF-2: immunoglobulin transcription factor 2
ITT: intent-to-treat
ITT analysis: intention-to-treat analysis
LCPUFAs: long-chain polyunsaturated fatty acids
n-3 LC-PUFAs: n-3 long-chain polyunsaturated fatty acids
LRTI: lower respiratory tract infections
MAOI: monoamine oxidase inhibitors
MDD: major depressive disorder
MED: minimum effective dose
MHC: major histocompatibility complex
NGS: next-generation sequencing
NMR spectra: nuclear magnetic resonance spectra
MRI scans: magnetic resonance imaging scans
MTHFRD: methylenetetrahydrofolate reductase deficiency
ODs: other dementias
PANSS: positive and negative syndrome scale

PFC: prefrontal cortex
PFC glia: prefrontal cortex glia
PFC/ACC: prefrontal cortex/anterior cingulate cortex
PUFA: polyunsaturated fatty acids
omega-3 PUFAs: ω-3 polyunsaturated fatty acids
RAD-seq: restriction-site-associated DNA sequencing
RBC: red blood cell
RBC membrane: red blood cell membrane
RCT: randomized, double-blind, placebo-controlled, parallel-group single-center, six month, augmentation trial
RR: relative risk
RRLs: reduced-representation libraries
RTD: ready to drink
SANS: scale for the assessment of negative symptoms
SNRI: serotonin-norepinephrine reuptake inhibitor
SQ: symptom questionnaire
SSRIs: selective serotonin reuptake inhibitors
TB: tuberculosis
TCF-4: transcription factor 4
TPUFAs: total polyunsaturated fatty acids
UFAs: unsaturated fatty acids
ω-3UFAs: omega-3 unsaturated fatty acids
undifferentiated UFAs: undifferentiated unsaturated fatty acids
WHO: World Health Organization
ZNF804A: Zinc finger protein 804A

1. INTRODUCTION

1.1. Concept of Nutraceuticals

Recently the term "nutraceuticals" has been used in the region of the functions of mainly phytochemicals and marine components. In 1989 the word nutraceuticals was coined from nutrition and pharmaceuticals [1].

On the difference between *functional food* and *nutraceutical*, Dr. Ekta Kalra of Nagpur College of Pharmacy, Maharashtra Nagpur University, India proposed in 2003 that *functional food* provides the required amounts, such as vitamins, fats, proteins, carbohydrates, and others essential for healthy survival of the human body. On the other hand, when *functional food* aids in prevention and/or treatment of disease(s) and/or disorder(s) other than anemia, it is called a *nutraceutical* [2].

It seems that nutraceuticals are the general food products derived from all natural food sources (mainly, phytochemicals and marine components) including three major nutrients and minor nutrients such as vitamins and minerals useful in obesity prevention or obesity amelioration and health maintenance. Therefore, nutraceutical substances are all foods or parts of a food that not only provide medical and medicinal benefits or health benefits by nutritionally and functionally excellent foods using food materials rich in nutrients, but also contribute in the prevention and treatment of diverse diseases [3].

Moreover, other definitions have been described of *nutraceuticals* [4-9] or *pharmaceuticals,* which originates from a newly coined word from farm and pharmaceuticals [10], and their health effects on human.

Based on the above definitions, nutraceuticals might be nearly divided into four parts: *functional foods* such as unsaturated fatty acid foods, color foods (carotene foods, flavonoid foods) and probiotic foods, *dietary supplements (nutritional supplements)* such as vitamin and mineral supplements, herbal supplements such as Ayurvedic herbal extracts, plant extracts and plant protein supplements like protein powder and healthy living lifestyle products, *functional beverages* such as sports drinks and fortified juices, energy drinks, ready to drink (RTD) teas, enhanced fruit drinks, soy beverages, and enhanced water, and *natural pharmaceuticals* such as a natural substance derived antibacterial agent, and discoloration and oxidation inhibitors for food derived from natural products [11]. This chapter describes the components and effects of nutraceutical antioxidants with diverse diseases including prevention and treatments against dementia, diabetes, and arthrosis.

2. Adjuvant Effect of Nutraceuticals as CAMs with Depression and Schizophrenia

2.1. Dietary Components against Depression

By the most important disease and injury trends since 1950 in nine cause-of-death clusters from the World Health Organization (WHO), it has been estimated that leading causes of disability-adjusted life years (DALYs) were ischaemic heart disease (IHD) at the highest probability, followed by unipolar major depression or major depressive disorder (MDD), road-traffic accidents, cerebrovascular disease, chronic obstructive pulmonary disease (COPD), lower respiratory tract infections (LRTI), tuberculosis (TB), war injuries, diarrheal diseases, and human immunodeficiency virus (HIV) or acquired immune deficiency syndrome (AIDS) virus. Unipolar major depression or MDD will become the second leading cause of disability worldwide by 2020, and unipolar major depression or MDD is second to ischemic heart disease. Additionally, unipolar major depression or MDD is becoming the leading cause in developing regions [12]. Based on these facts, by today, dietary supplements have been tried for prevention, improvement, and treatment against depression.

2.1.1. Omega-3 Fatty Acids

The efficacy of omega-3 highly unsaturated fatty acids (ω-3HUFAs) such as docosahexaenoic acid (DHA) (Figure 1) and eicosapentaenoic acid (EPA) (Figure 1) derived from α-linolenic acid (Figure 1), and omega-6 fatty acids in the depressive patients has been mostly focused in treatment of depressive symptoms in both unipolar depression and bipolar depression among mood disorders [13].

The (g/100 g) ω-3UFAs are in vegetables, fruits, and nuts. Seeds, flaxseed: 22.813 for 18:3 undifferentiated UFAs including α-linolenic acid (ALA) of 28.730 total polyunsaturated fatty acids (TPUFAs); oil, walnut: 10.400 for 18:3 undifferentiated UFAs of 63.300 TPUFAs; oil, olive, salad or cooking: 0.761 for 18:3 undifferentiated UFAs of 10.523 TPUFAs; beans, kidney, all types, mature seeds, raw: 0.279 for 18:3 undifferentiated UFAs of 0.457 TPUFAs; soybeans, mature seeds, raw: 1.330 for 18:3 undifferentiated UFAs of 11.255 TPUFAs; spinach, raw: 0.138 for 18:3 undifferentiated UFAs of 0.165 TPUFAs; brussels sprouts, raw: 0.099 for 18:3 undifferentiated UFAs of 0.153 TPUFAs; bananas, raw: 0.027 for 18:3 undifferentiated UFAs of 0.073 TPUFAs; grapes, American type (slip skin), raw: 0.024 for 18:3 undifferentiated UFAs of 0.102 TPUFAs; cauliflower, raw: 0.015 for 18:3 undifferentiated UFAs and 0.015 for ALA, of 0.031 TPUFAs; chestnuts, Japanese, raw: 0.013 for 18:3 undifferentiated UFAs of 0.138 TPUFAs; cucumber, with peel, raw: 0.005 for 18:3 undifferentiated UFAs of 0.032 TPUFAs; tomatoes, red, ripe, raw, year round average: 0.003 for 18:3 undifferentiated UFAs of 0.083 TPUFAs; peaches, yellow, raw: 0.002 for 18:3 undifferentiated UFAs of 0.086 TPUFAs. Among the above common daily foods, seeds (flaxseed); oil (walnut); and olive, salad, or cooking oil especially are richer in UFAs including ω-3HUFAs compared to UFAs in other foods [14].

In 2006 a group from the Regulatory Policies Laboratory, Mario Negri Institute for Pharmacological Research, Milan, Italy, reviewed the role of marine n-3 long-chain polyunsaturated fatty acids (n-3 LC-PUFAs) such as EPA and DHA and their derivatives such as ethyl eicosapentaenoic acid (E-EPA) (Figure 2) in brain functions including development of the central nervous system (CNS) and neurological disorders, excepting ALA from the analysis, because of its vegetable origin. It is known that ~50%–60% (dry weight) of the adult brain is composed of lipids, and among these ~50%–60% lipids, ~35% are phospholipids containing mainly two LC-PUFAs such as arachidonic acid (AA) (Figure 2) and DHA with their highest contents [15]. However, humans and animals cannot synthesize these highly UFAs inside their bodies. Humans and animals must ingest these UFAs from the outside. Therefore these UFAs have been treated as essential fatty acids (EFAs).

The principal dietary source of n-6 LC-PUFA is LA (Figure 2). An n-6 LC-PUFA LA is mostly found in vegetable oils, whereas n-3 LC-PUFA ALA is abundantly the natural precursor of n-3 LC-PUFA in green-leaved plants. Two n-3 LC-PUFAs DHA and EPA which are the most abundant and important n-3 LC-PUFAs of the CNS, are mainly found in sea fish [16, 17].

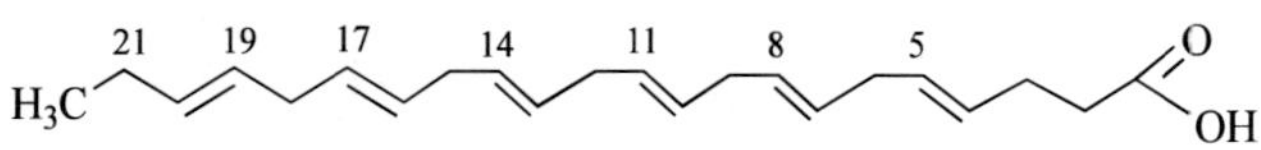

docosahexaenoic acid (DHA. 22:6n3. C22:6(ω-3). 22:6n3. **1**)

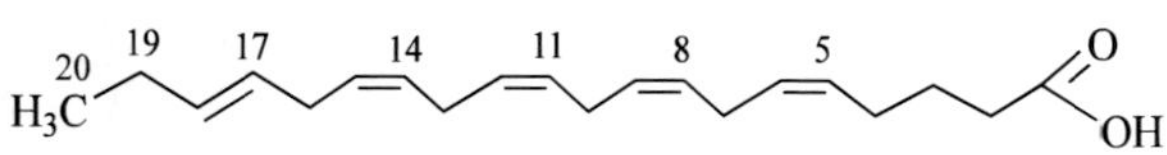

eicosapentaenoic acid (EPA. C20:5(ω-3). 20:5n3. **2**)

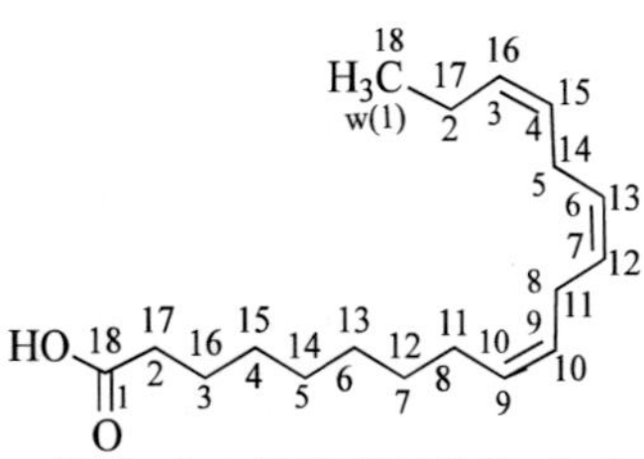

α-linolenic acid ((9,12,15)-linolenic acid, 18:3(9,12,15) acid, C18:3, ω-3, **3**)

Figure 1. Docosahexaenoic acid (DHA. 22:6n3. C22:6(ω-3). 22:6n3. **1**), eicosapentaenoic acid (EPA. C20:5(ω-3). 20:5n3. **2**), and α-linolenic acid (linolenic acid. ALA. 18:3(n-3), 18:3($\Delta^{9,12,15}$), 18:3n3. **3**).

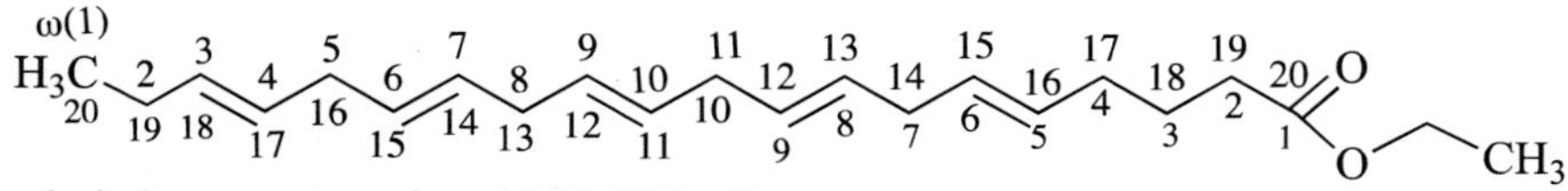

ethyl eicosapentaenoic acid (E-EPA. **4**)

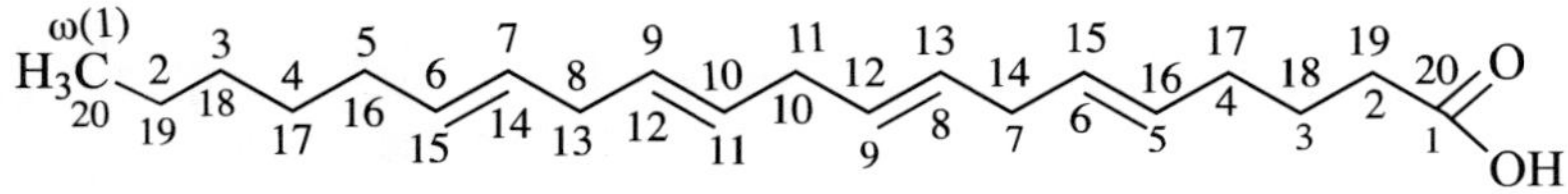

arachidonic acid (AA. C20:4(ω-6). 20:4n6. **5**)

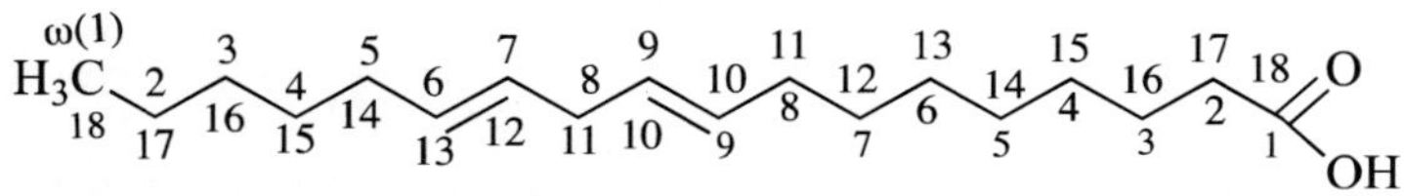

linoleic acid (LA, 18:2n6(ω-6). **6**)

Figure 2. Ethyl eicosapentaenoic acid (E-EPA. **4**), arachidonic acid (AA. C20:4(ω-6). 20:4n6. **5**) and linoleic acid (LA, 18:2n6(ω-6). **6**).

2.1.1.1. Relationship between CSF 5-HIAA and Cholesterol Lowering

There exists a significant association between low 5-hydroxyindoleacetic acid (5-HIAA) (Figure 3) concentrations in cerebrospinal fluid (CSF) and increased risk of attempted and completed suicide in biological psychiatry [18, 19].

The low 5-HIAA concentrations in CSF of an indicator of reduced serotonin (Figure 3) turnover rate in the frontal cortex [20] was also associated with impaired impulse control [21], unprovoked violent behavior and aggressive behavior [22], and hostility [23]. It is also known that mortality due to suicide, homicide, and trauma appears to increase in therapeutic trials designed to lower plasma cholesterol [24].

From the above decreases of two biological components such as *both* the low 5-HIAA concentrations in CSF *and* the lowering of plasma cholesterol, Dr. Engelberg proposed that lowering plasma cholesterol may be a trigger to cause decrease of 5-HIAA concentrations in CSF [25]. When plasma cholesterol levels were lowered by reducing cholesterol intake, rhesus monkeys became more aggressive, while 5-HIAA concentrations in CSF were also reduced [26].

In 1986 a group from the Section of Analytical Chemistry, Laboratory of Clinical Studies, DICBR, National Institute of Alcohol Abuse and Alcoholism, showed that DHA is selectively concentrated in neuronal membranes and appears critical for proper neuronal function [27, 28].

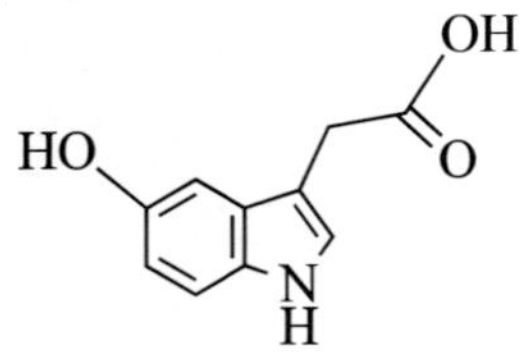

5-hydroxyindoleacetic acid (5-HIAA. **7**)

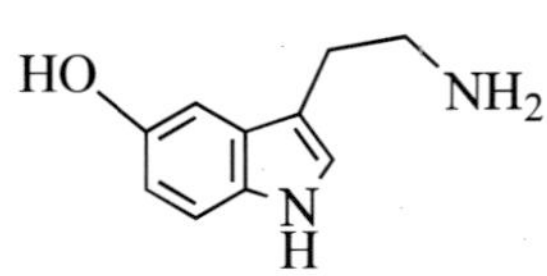

serotonin (5HT, 5-hydroxytryptamine. **8**)

Figure 3. 5-Hydroxyindoleacetic acid (5-HIAA. **7**) and serotonin (5HT, 5-hydroxytryptamine. **8**).

2.1.1.2. Relationship between CSF 5-HIAA and Omega-3 Fatty Acids

There is novel evidence on the risk of attempted and completed suicide in biological psychiatry that plasma concentrations of polyunsaturated EFAs might participate more closely in CSF 5-HIAA concentrations compared to plasma cholesterol concentrations as follows: In 1987 a group from the Forensic Psychiatric Department, Helsinki University Central Hospital, Finland showed for the first time that low plasma cholesterol concentrations among violent offenders means lack of EFA DHA and docosapentaenoic acid (DPA) (Figure 4) [29].

In 1992 a group from the Department of Biochemistry, University Department of Child Health, Royal Hospital for Sick Children, Yorkhill, Glasgow, UK confirmed that supplementation of formula milks that contains a UFA DHA for term infants and supplementation of formula milks with two UFAs such as both DHA and AA for preterm infants were beneficial to promotion of their subsequent neurodevelopment and function. This means that diets with insufficient DHA decreased DHA concentration in the human brain [30].

Plasma DHA concentrations were negatively correlated with CSF 5-HIAA concentrations among an independent group of both subjects for their history of violent behavior and impulsive behavior and control subjects having a history of nonviolent and nonimpulsive behavior [19].

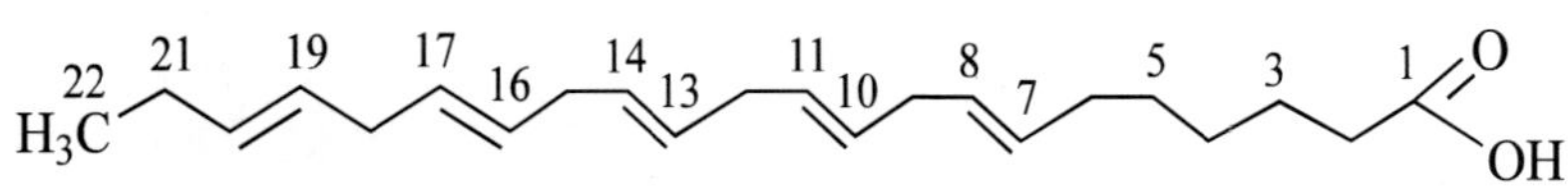

docosapentaenoic acid (DPA. 22:5n3. C22:5(ω-3). **9**)

Figure 4. Docosapentaenoic acid (DPA. 22:5n3. C22:5(ω-3). **9**).

Based on the above facts, in 1998 a group from the Laboratory of Membrane Biochemistry and Biophysics, National Institute on Alcohol Abuse and Alcoholism tried to replicate the negative correlation between plasma DHA and CSF 5-HIAA in a second observational study of an independent group of subjects selected for their history of 27 (male 21 and female 6) violent, impulsive behaviors and in a set of 31 (male 22 and female 9) nonviolent control subjects, measuring CSF 5-HIAA and HVA (Figure 5), fasting total cholesterol, and plasma fatty acid concentrations in violent subjects and nonviolent subjects matched for severity of alcohol dependence. HVA is a major catecholamine metabolite used as a reagent to detect oxidative enzymes and is associated with dopamine levels in the brain.

First, from analysis of variance comparisons of violent and nonviolent groups on concentrations (pmol/mL cell) of CSF 5-HIAA, the violent subjects (72 pmol/mL cell) were significantly lower compared to the nonviolent (95 pmol/mL cell) subjects. Second, on the score of Buss Durkee Hostility Inventory (Buss Durkee Score), the violent subjects (Buss Durkee Score: 45) showed a significantly higher score compared to the nonviolent (Buss Durkee Score: 20) subjects.

Third, on the Brown Goodwin Lifetime History of Aggression Scale (Brown Goodwin Score), the violent subjects (Brown Goodwin Score: 20) showed a significantly higher score compared to the nonviolent (Brown Goodwin Score: 12) subjects. The violent subjects had a significantly higher lifetime violence rating and hostility ratings and lower concentrations of CSF 5-HIAA compared to nonviolent subjects.

Second, on alcohol-related variables and neurotransmitter metabolites, the groups did not differ in age, quantitative measures of alcohol consumption, or indices of alcohol-related liver damage. These measures might have been a confounding factor in the relationship between plasma lipids and CSF neurotransmitter metabolites. Third, in plasma fatty acid composition, there were no differences in concentrations of any individual fatty acid or total plasma cholesterol between the violent subjects and the nonviolent subjects.

Fourth, in concentrations of CSF 5-HIAA, the violent subjects had significantly lower concentrations of CSF 5-HIAA compared to the nonviolent subjects. Plasma DHA was negatively correlated with CSF 5-HIAA only among violent subjects.

In conclusion, intake of essential fatty acids such as DHA contained in daily foods may change neurotransmitter concentrations. It will be neccessary to confirm that increasing dietary intake of DHA will influence the increase or decrease of either CSF 5-HIAA concentrations or impulsive behavior and violent behavior, by using dietary intervention trials including the epidemiological survey [31].

Based on a hypothesis that lack of ω–3 fatty acid (ω-3 PUFAs or n-3 PUFAs) is aetiologically serious in depression, with DHA belonging to the ω-3 PUFA family being a crucial component of synaptic cell membranes, in 1998, a group from the University Department of Psychiatry, University of Sheffield, UK measured ω-3 fatty acid levels in red blood cell (RBC) membrane in a group of 10 depressed patients and 14 healthy control subjects. The depressed patients showed significant depletion of the RBC membrane ω-3 PUFAs caused by reduced calorie intake. Severity of depression correlated *both* with the number having a negative value on RBC membrane ω-3 PUFA levels *and* with dietary intake of ω-3 PUFA levels compared to those (both the number having a negative value on RBC membrane ω-3 PUFA levels *and* dietary intake of ω-3 PUFA levels) of healthy control subjects.

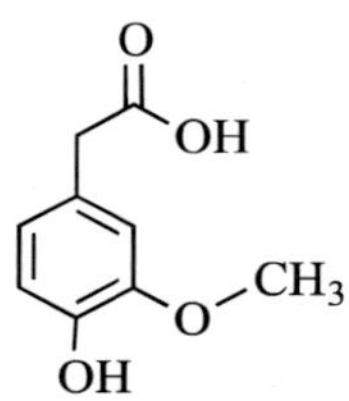

homovanillic acid (HVA. **10**)

Figure 5. Homovanillic acid (HVA. **10**).

Results suggest that lower RBC membrane ω-3 PUFA levels are highly associated with severity of depression. At the same time, a possibility was clinically shown that depressive symptoms could be lessened by supplementation of ω-3 PUFAs [32, 33].

2.1.1.3. Effects of ω-3 Fatty Acid Derivative E-EPA as an Adjunct to Antidepressant Treatment

There are epidemiological relationships between ingestion of ω-3 fatty acids in fish oil and low rates of depressive disorder [34]. In 1999 a group from Brigham and Women's Hospital, Department of Psychiatry, Harvard Medical School confirmed that a controlled, double-blind trial represented significant therapeutic efficacy without the side effects of ω-3 fatty acids in prevention of bipolar manic-depressive illness, given results by administration of supplied ω-3 fatty acids (9.6 g/day) vs. placebo (olive oil) in usual treatment for 30 patients with bipolar disorder during four months [35]. This means that ω-3 fatty acids have an effect on CSF 5-hydroxytryptamine (serotonin) metabolites [31]. In 1998 a group from the University Department of Psychiatry, University of Sheffield, UK confirmed that changes in fatty acid levels in the daily diet and RBCs of depressed patients and lower RBC membrane ω-3 fatty acids, especially lower DHA of a crucial component of synaptic cell membranes, are associated with severity of depression [32]. In 1999 a group from University Department of Psychiatry, Clinical Research Center for Mental Health, Antwerp, Belgium observed changes in serum fatty acid composition in depressive disorder along with abnormal metabolism of ω-3FAc. They also observed alterations of fatty acid from abnormal metabolism in depression related to inflammatory response. Therefore if serum fatty acid composition could not be improved, the disorder might continue in spite of administration of an effective antidepressant such as a selective serotonin reuptake inhibitor (SSRI), serotonin modulator, or serotonin stimulator [36]. In 1999 it was proposed that ω-3FAcs are the mechanistic "missing link" connecting cardiovascular disease and depressive disorder, representing a key pathophysiological clue to the mechanism of depressive disorder [37].

Based on the above facts, in 2002 a group from the Ministry of Health Mental Health Center, Faculty of Health Sciences, Ben Gurion University of the Negev, Beer-Sheva, Israel studied effects of ω-3 FA derivative E-EPA (derived from 96% pure fish oil) as an adjunct to antidepressant treatment for episodes of depressive disorder in 20 patients with recurrent unipolar depressive disorder who were receiving maintenance antidepressant therapy. Fish oil was stabilized with 0.2% vitamin E (Figure 6) in 500 mg soft gelatin capsules/day. The ω-3FAc derivative E-EPA or matching placebo was administered by oral administration in 1 g doses twice a day for a total of 2 g/day.

On the effects of E-EPA or placebo for treatment of depressive episodes in 20 depressant patients receiving maintenance antidepressant medication, using the Hamilton rating scale for depression (HRSD), treatment and time showed a statistically significant interaction. The effect of E-EPA showed a significant difference from the effect of placebo after around Week 2.

Second, even accepting the patients who dropped out of the study, there exists from HRSD values a statistically significant interaction between E-EPA treatment and time (Weeks 1 to 4). Mean reduction in the Hamilton depression scale score (HDSS) in depressant patients receiving E-EPA was 12.4 points compared to HDSS 1.6 points in depressant patients receiving placebo for four weeks. This means that significant reduction by oral administration of E-EPA was clinically effective for improvement of depression, because 6 of 10 (60%) depressant patients receiving E-EPA showed remarkable effectiveness while only 1 of 10 (10%) depressant patients receiving placebo showed a 50% reduction in the HDSS. The effect of E-EPA was significant from Week 2 of administration, similar to the time course for effectiveness of antidepressant drugs such as citalopram, fluoxetine, fluvoxamine, mirtazapine, moclobemide, and paroxetine (Figure 6).

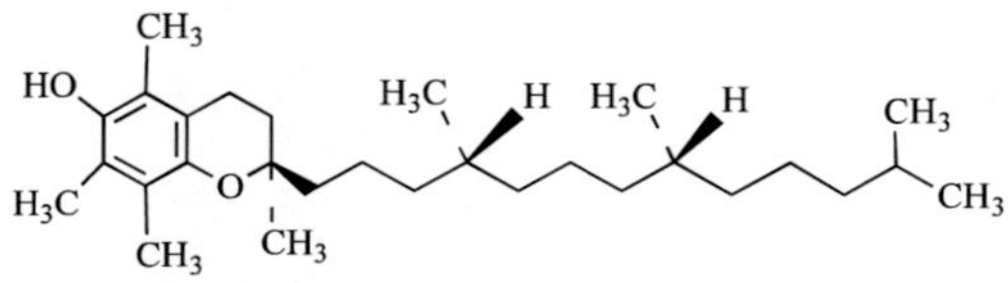

α-tocopherol (vitamin E. **11**)

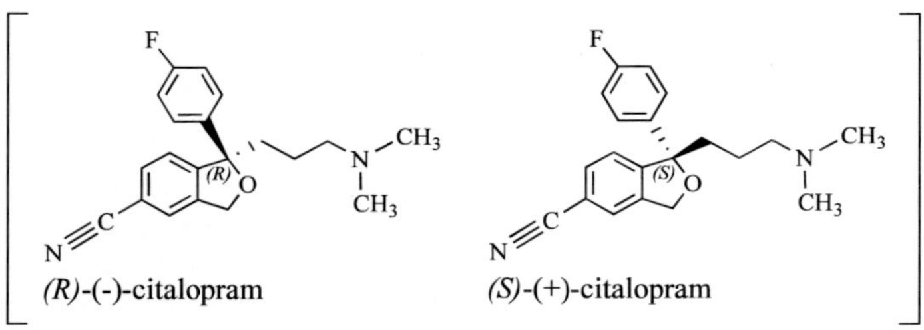

citalopram (**12**)

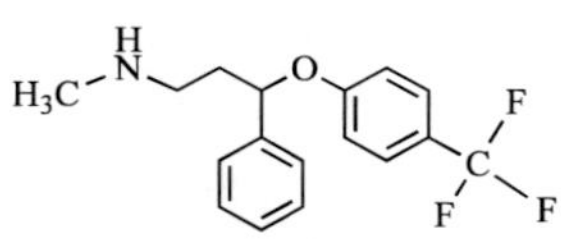

fluoxetine (**13**)

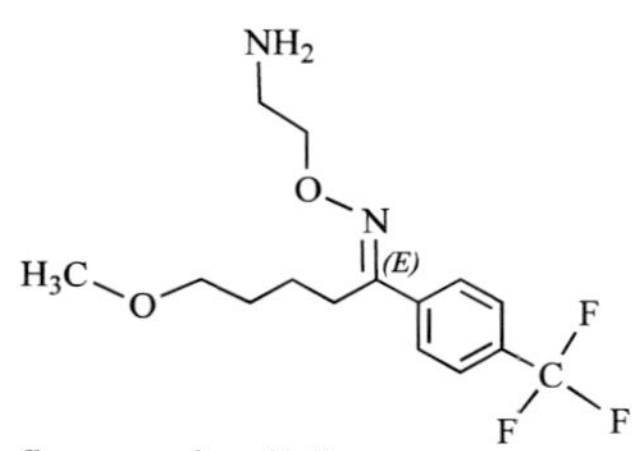

fluvoxamine (**14**)

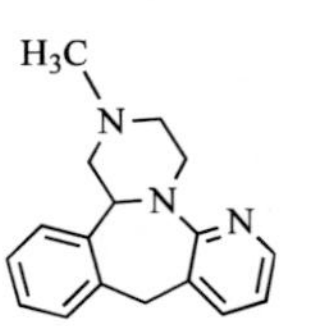

mirtazapine (**15**)

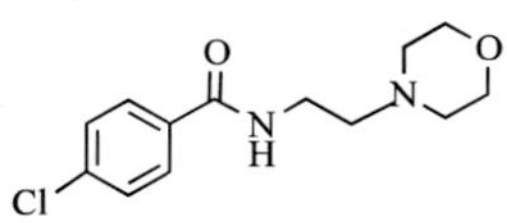

moclobemide (**16**)

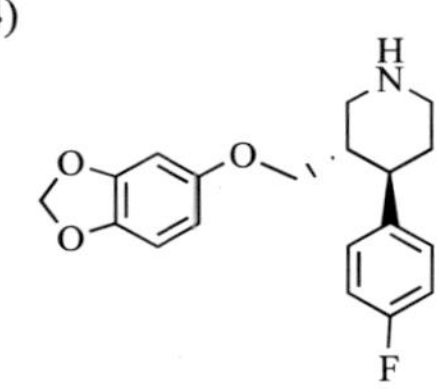

paroxetine (**17**)

Figure 6. α-Tocopherol (vitamin E. **11**), citalopram (**12**), fluoxetine (**13**), fluvoxamine (**14**), mirtazapine (**15**), moclobemide (**16**) and paroxetine (**17**).

These results suggest that E-EPA had an effect against core depressive symptoms such as depressed mood, guilt feelings, and worthlessness, as well as insomnia [33, 38].

2.1.1.4. Improvement Effect of ω-3 Fatty Acids for MDD

In 2003 a group from the Department of Psychiatry, China Medical College Hospital, Taichung, Taiwan conducted an eight-week, preliminary double-blind, placebo-controlled trial to examine effects of administration of two omega-3 PUFAs such as DHA and EPA in a top dosage (9.6 g/day) in the usual treatment on improvement of MDD, using 28 major depressive disorder patients over 18 with the 21-item version of the Hamilton rating scale for depression ($HRSD_{21}$). Preadministration psychiatric status and postadministration clinical outcome were evaluated with $HRSD_{21}$ [39]. Each capsule of omega-3 fatty acid concentrate from the body oil of menhaden fish contains 440 mg of EPA and 220 mg of DHA.

There were no statistical differences on demographics, clinical characteristics, or omega-3 PUFAs composition in the RBC membrane based on the Mann–Whitney *U*-test. Each participant in a group of 12 patients who received omega-3 PUFA treatment (ω3)—or 10 placebo patients—was free from medications such as fluvoxamine, trazodone (Figure 7) or moclobemide. The subjects of both groups receiving these medications were converted into fluoxetine equivalents.

Second, the difference in $HRSD_{21}$ score between the omega-3 group (score: -2.5) and the placebo group (score: -2.5) began after one week: the $HRSD_{21}$ score was around -6.0 for the omega-3 group and around -4.0 for the placebo group at two weeks, around -8.0 for the omega-3 group and around -4.5 for the placebo group at four weeks, around -13.0 for the omega-3 group and around -4.0 for the placebo group at six weeks, and around -14.0 for the omega-3 group and around -6.0 for the placebo group at eight weeks, respectively.

From the results, the $HRSD_{21}$ score of subjects in the omega-3 group showed significant differences from the fourth week after administration of omega-3 PUFA treatment (ω3). The ratio of reducing total $HRSD_{21}$ score in the omega-3 group was significantly much higher compared to total $HRSD_{21}$ score in the placebo group.

Third, regarding the effect of omega-3 PUFA and placebo supplement on fatty acid composition in RBC membrane, the mean posttreatment value of DHA to depressive patients in the omega-3 group was significantly much higher than the mean posttreatment value of DHA in the period of pretreatment. However, the mean posttreatment value of EPA to depressive patients in the omega-3 group is not significantly different from that in the period of pre-treatment. Additionally, there is no significant difference between pre-treatment levels and posttreatment levels of DHA or EPA for subjects in the placebo group.

These results suggest that the deficiency of DHA is more prominent and serious compared to deficiency of EPA. EPA exists with a very small quantity in neuronal membranes, while DHA is a major constituent of the neuronal membrane phospholipid with the important functioning of neurotransmitters including the dopaminergic pathway and serotonergic pathway [19, 31, 34, 38, 40, 41].

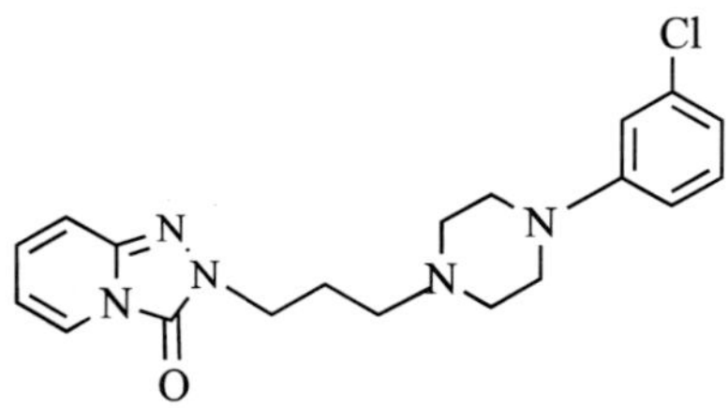

trazodone (**18**)

Figure 7. Trazodone (**18**).

2.1.1.5. Improvement Effect of DPA, DHA, LA, and AA with Schizophrenia

The improvement factor by administration of PUFA in schizophrenia is shown in many studies, without showing definite variation on improvement of schizophrenics. In 2013 a group from the Mentrum Institute for Mental Health, Amsterdam, the Netherlands examined epidemiologically PUFAs measured in RBCs and schizophrenia, using a systematic review and meta-analysis for DPA, DHA, LA, and AA.

First, comparison of PUFA content in the erythrocyte cell membrane between schizophrenics and healthy volunteers (controls) was made using 18 studies with 642 patients (169 were antipsychotic-naïve) and 574 controls. As a result, suggestive evidence was confirmed that levels of DPA and DHA showed decrease both in patients currently being treated with antipsychotic medication and antipsychotic-naïve patients compared to levels of DPA and DHA for healthy volunteers (controls).

Second, it suggests that levels of LA showed decreases in the antipsychotic subgroup (low administration group of antipsychotic) compared to levels of LA of schizophrenics. On the other hand, levels of LA did not show the decrease in the antipsychotic-naïve group compared to levels of LA of schizophrenics. Third, antipsychotic-naïve patients decreased most convincingly in levels of AA.

These results show substantial evidence that decreased levels of DPA, DHA, and AA are associated with the schizophrenia syndrome, in addition to a possible influence of antipsychotic administration. Because these results showed large heterogeneity (the quality of being diverse and not comparable in kind), these conclusions should be investigated more deeply from a standpoint of the mechanism between PUFAs and antipsychotics [42].

2.1.1.6. Synergistic Effect of EPA + DHA for First-Episode Schizophrenia

It is known that schizophrenia is a neurodevelopmental disorder and a neurodegenerative disorder displaying disturbance in multiple neuro-transmission pathways. Given that PUFAs are essential for maintenance of normal neurodevelopment, metabolic disturbance of PUFAs might be involved in the etiology of neurodevelopmental disorders such as schizophrenia, including both positive symptom of hallucination and delusion, and negative symptoms of autism and flat affect [17, 43]. PUFAs are significantly rich in the CNS and these PUFAs in the CNS are the main constituents of neuronal membrane phospholipids. The two most abundant LCPUFAs in the brain are DHA and AA. LCPUFAs such as DHA and AA are incorporated as SN2 docosahexaenoate or SN2 arachidonate in the Sn-2 position of phospholipids, respectively. Both DHA and AA are released from membrane phospholipids by phospholipase A2, and two released derivatives such as both DHA and AA take part in neuronal impulse transmission. Neuronal membranes are rich in DHA and DHA essential for normal brain development.

The balance of the DHA/AA (n-3/n-6) ratio is important in maintenance of an appropriate level of membrane fluidity. Especially, this means that the balance of DHA/AA ratio is essential for ion channel function, membrane receptor activity, and release of neurohormones, such as the signaling processes of every cell on risk of cognitive decline. The numerous neurotransmission pathways have been found to be dysfunctional in schizophrenia. It is thought that membrane phospholipids modulate activity of both receptors and are involved in signal transduction as part of the etiology of schizophrenia [45, 46].

The following facts also are known on n-3 PUFA and schizophrenia: On the efficacy of n-3 PUFA in schizophrenia, n-3 PUFA supplementation studies in schizophrenia suggests that intervention with n-3 PUFA can be more effective when n-3 PUFA is administered at the initial symptom of schizophrenia compared to PUFA administration after midterm symptom of schizophrenia [47-53]. Second, on PUFA and the reduced risk of adverse effects such as tardive dyskinesia and metabolic side effects associated with antipsychotics, the reduction in the intensity of side effects of antipsychotics associated with n-3 PUFA supplementation can increase adherence to antipsychotics, and subsequently give favorable effects to improving severity of symptoms and the relapse rate in the first episode of schizophrenia [54-61].

Second, on relapse in schizophrenia, these observations have caused interest in relapse prevention for schizophrenia and have prompted repeated attempts to understand risk factors responsible for recurrence of psychotic exacerbation [47-53]. Third, on relapse risk factors, it is reported that both relapse duration and treatment intensity depend on brain tissue loss; but while treatment effects are more diffusely distributed, relapse effects are most strongly associated with changes to frontal lobe tissue. It was concluded that relapse prevention should be sustained using the lowest possible medication dosages to control the schizophrenia symptom [51, 53, 62, 63]. Fourth, on n-3 PUFA in relapse prevention, in 2014 a group from the Department of Psychiatry, Faculty of Medicine and Health Sciences, Stellenbosch University, Cape Town, South Africa concluded that n-3 PUFAs + ALA does not appear to be a suitable alternative to maintenance of antipsychotic treatment in relapse prevention. The group showed that current treatment guidelines suggesting antipsychotic discontinuation two to three years after the first psychotic episode should be revised on the basis of their findings [64]. Fifth, regarding rationale for the study on schizophrenia and n-3 PUFA, it was suggested that DHA plays a unique role in neurodevelopment [65, 66], prevention of neuropsychiatric disorder, [67] and neurodegenerative disorder [68, 69].

In 2015, proving the synergistic effect of EPA + DHA, a group from the Department of Affective and Psychotic Disorders, Medical University of Lodz, Lodz, Poland conducted three administrations of a long-term, randomized, placebo-controlled, single dose treatment of EPA + DHA. The intervention in the first-questionnaire was with eight out of nine schizophrenia patients, including a baseline visit (control) and omega-3 fatty acids in first-episode schizophrenia. The randomized, controlled study of efficacy and relapse prevention (OFFER) study aims to systematically evaluate long-term efficacy of n-3 PUFA in reducing the psychopathological symptom and preventing relapse in patients with first-episode schizophrenia. In this study, the participants were supplemented with 1,320 mg/day of EPA and 880 mg/day of DHA. Olive oil was used as placebo (control), because olive oil contains mainly monounsaturated fatty acids (MUFAs) and only small amounts of UFA and PUFA. Generally, the intervention period in assessing the efficacy of n-3 PUFA in schizophrenia lasted 8 to 12 weeks. No longer-term trials were conducted. The group study was planned to last 52 weeks of the intervention period and contained two phases, intervention and follow-up. The intervention period was continued for 26 weeks. The schizophrenia patients were observed for the 26 weeks after the intervention phase.

A randomized, double-blind, placebo-controlled, parallel-group single-center, six-month, augmentation trial (RCT) of an intervention was based on 2.2 g of EPA + DHA added onto an adjustable dose of antipsychotic medication in first-episode schizophrenia patients. Especially, the outcome measure was focused on efficacy of n-3 PUFA in reducing severity of schizophrenia symptoms, by using the positive and negative syndrome scale (PANSS) for schizophrenia. Subsequently, the secondary outcome measures included two outcomes such as the *efficacy* of six-month add-on therapy with n-3 PUFA in reducing the risk of relapse in first-episode schizophrenia patients during the first year of therapy, and the *influence* of n-3 PUFA on depressive symptoms regarding general functioning and level of insight. In addition to the longitudinal design of the outcome measures, the study aimed to observe the relationship of the expected change, such as structural brain change observed in magnetic resonance imaging (MRI) scans, oxidative stress, and defense mechanisms, as well as brain plasticity [43].

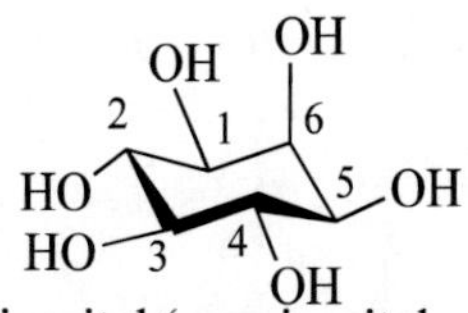

inositol (*myo*-inositol. vitamin B8. **19**)

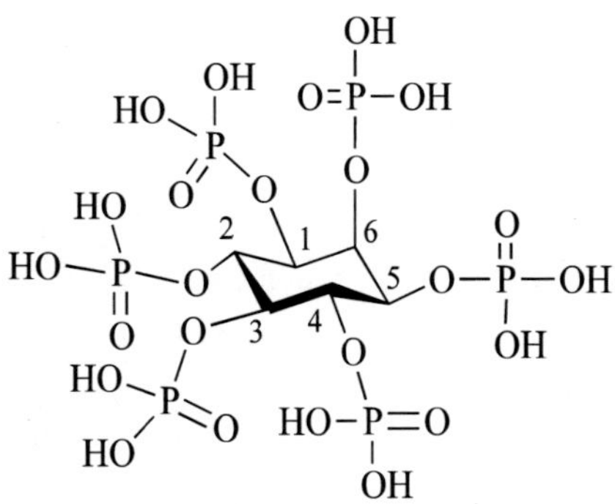

phytic acid (myo-inositol-1,2,3,4,5,6-hexaphosphate. **20**)

Figure 8. Inositol (*myo*-inositol. Vitamin B8. **19**) and phytic acid (myo-inositol-1,2,3,4,5,6-hexaphosphate. **20**).

2.1.2. Inositol

Inositol (former names *meso*-inositol or i-inositol) (Figure 8) is a sixfold alcohol (polyol) of cyclohexane. Inositol exists in nine possible stereoisomers, of which the most prominent form, widely occurring in nature, is phytic acid (Figure 8) or inositol [70].

Inositol is rich in fruits and vegetables. The phytic acid content (mg/100 g edible parts) of phytic acid containing fruits and nuts and seeds is as follows: 10 for avocado, average, 40 for dates, raw, 90 for dates, dried, 80 for dates, dried and weighed with stones, 30 for figs, dried, 30 for figs, ready to eat, 30 for mangoes, ripe raw, 20 for mangoes, raw, weighed with skin and stone, and 10 for raisins, respectively. Phytic acid content (mg/100 g edible parts) of nuts and seeds is 1,070 for almond, 400 for almond, weighed with shells, 1,090 for almond, toasted, 970 for cashew nuts, plain, 970 for cashew nuts, roasted and salted, 10 for chestnuts, 10 for chestnuts, weighed with shells, 20 for chestnuts, dried, 770 for peanuts, plain, 530 for peanuts, plain, weighed with shells, 680 for peanuts, dry roasted, 750 for peanuts, roasted and salted, 1,380 for sesame seeds, 3,000 for sunflower seeds, 3,110 for sunflower seeds, toasted, 580 for walnuts, and 250 for walnuts, weighed with shells [71, 72].

2.1.2.1. Inositol and Depression

Inositol has been used as a folklore remedy for neurasthenia and mild depression in Europe [73]. The level of inositol in CSF was lower compared to lthe evel of inositol for healthy persons [74].

In 1993 a group from the Division of Psychiatry and Abarbanel Mental Health Center, Tel Aviv University, Israel examined treatment-effective one-day dose of inositol. Inositol is an important precursor for second messenger synthesis and reduces by lithium treatment in both rat brain and in human CSF in depression. First, the open trial of 6 g inositol/day for 11 depressed patients resistant to previous treatment led to major improvement in 9 depressed patients. Enzyme synthesizing inositol was elevated in the schizophrenic patient, suggesting an attempted compensation for possible inositol deficiency. Second, a controlled, double-blind, crossover trial for 10 chronic schizophrenic patients of 6 g inositol/day for 30 days did not show any effectiveness. These results show ~82% positive improvement effect for the schizophrenic patient. Oral administration of 6 g inositol/day caused at times mild flatulence as the only side effect [75].

Based on this result, in 1995 the group from the Yehuda Abarbanel Mental Health Center, Bat Yam, Israel examined CSF levels of inositol in depressed patients, using a double-blind, controlled trial with 12 g inositol/day for 13 subjects or 12 g placebo/day for 15 control subjects administered to depressed patients for four weeks. Overall improvement in scores on the HRSD was significantly greater for inositol compared to overall improvement of placebo at Week 4. Moreover, kidney or liver function change could not be observed from a hematological point of view. The results show that the double-blind, controlled trial using inositol may be the first use of inositol as the precursor strategy for a second messenger rather than a neurotransmitter in depression treatment. While inositol showed a significant antidepressant effect, further repetitive experiments are important in order to accumulate further evidence [76, 77].

2.1.2.2. Improvement Effect for Panic Disorder with Inositol

In 1995 a group from the Soroka Medical Center, Kupat Holim Sick Fund of the Histadrut, Israel examined the effectiveness of inositol against panic disorder. First, 21 panic disorder patients with or without agoraphobia completed a double-blind, placebo-controlled, four-week, random-assignment crossover treatment trial of inositol 12 g/day. Second, both frequency and severity of panic attacks and severity of agoraphobia showed significantly more reductions with minimal side effects after inositol administration compared to frequency and severity after placebo (control) administration. Results show that inositol is effective and safe, with side effects in a range that can be almost ignored for panic disorder patients. Therefore, the greatest feature of inositol is being a naturally derived ingredient contained in human daily diets and at the same time being one of the nutraceuticals for prevention and treatment of panic disorder patients [78].

2.1.2.3. Improvement Effect for Depression with Inositol

In 1997 a group from the Ministry of Health Mental Health Center, Faculty of Health Sciences, Ben Gurion University of the Negev, Israel performed controlled trials of inositol in psychiatry. Inositol is a simple polyol precursor in a second messenger system important in the brain, and inositol in CSF decreases depression significantly. A double-blind, controlled trial was performed with oral administration of 12 g inositol daily using 28 depressed patients over four weeks. The inositol administration group showed significantly better overall improvement without changes of hematology function, kidney or liver functions compared to the overall improvement effect of the control group after four weeks, using the HDSS.

Second, because diverse antidepressants are effective for panic disorder patients, 21 panic disorder patients with or without agoraphobia of the 28 depressed patients completed both a double-blind, placebo-controlled trial and random-assignment crossover treatment trial using oral administration of 12 g inositol/day over four weeks. The frequency and severity of panic attacks and severity of agoraphobia in the inositol administered group showed significantly more decrease, with negligible side effects compared to frequency and severity of the control group. SSRIs and serotonin were beneficial for treatment of OCD, and inositol can reverse desensitization with serotonin receptors.

Thirteen OCD patients completed a double-blind, controlled, crossover trial of an 18 g inositol administered group or placebo control for six weeks, respectively. Oral administration of inositol reduced significantly scores of OCD symptoms compared to scores of the placebo control, using HRSD. Fourth, a controlled, double-blind, crossover trial of 12 g inositol daily for a month using 12 anergic schizophrenic patients did not show any beneficial effects. Fifth, when a double-blind, controlled, crossover trial of 6 g inositol daily vs. glucose (Figure 9) for one month was carried out in 11 AD patients, the administered group of 6 g inositol daily showed apparently better overall therapeutic effect compared to the overall therapeutic effect of the 6 g glucose daily administered group.

Sixth, antidepressant drugs can improve ADD or ADHD with hyperactive symptomatology. Oral administration of inositol in children with ADD or ADHD in a double-blind, crossover, placebo-controlled manner was carried out. Inosotol 200 mg/kg body weight was orally administered to 11 children (mean age 8.9 ± 3.6 years) in the inositol group or the placebo (control) group during an eight-week trial. Oral administration of inositol showed a trend of aggravation with ADD or ADHD compared to aggravation with oral administration of the placebo (control) group. SSRIs and serotonin are helpful in at least some symptoms of autism. However, this controlled, double-blind, crossover trial of inositol 200 mg/kg/day showed no benefit in nine children with autism.

Cholinergic agonists improve ECT induced memory impairment. Inositol metabolism is involved in the second messenger system for several muscarinic cholinergic receptors. Inositol 6 g daily was given by oral administration in a crossover double-blind manner for five days before the fifth or sixth ECT to a series of 12 memory-impaired patients; however, effect of inositol was not observed after the fifth or sixth ECT.

Results of these six experiments reveal therapeutic effects for the spectrum of illness responsive to SSRIs or serotonin, such as depression, panic syndrome, and OCD. On the other hand, inositol reveals no therapeutic effects for schizophrenia, AD, ADD or ADHD, autism, or ECT-induced cognitive impairment [79].

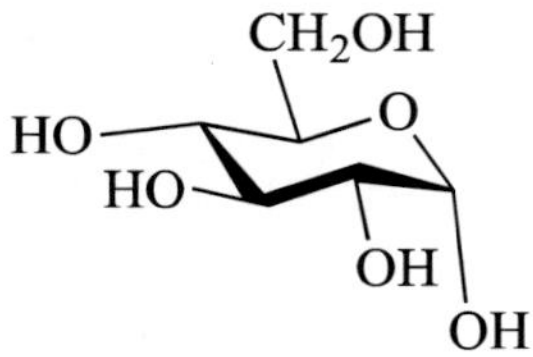

D(+)-glucose (**21**)

Figure 9. D(+)-Glucose (**21**).

2.1.2.4. Selective Serotonin Reuptake Inhibition of Inositol

In 1999 a group from the Ministry of Health Mental Health Center, Faculty of Health Sciences, Ben Gurion University of the Negev, Israel examined combined administration of inositol, serotonin, and SSRIs in treatment of depression. First, 27 depressed patients completed a double-blind, controlled, four-week trial by two combined administration methods of either SSRIs or serotonin + placebo or SSRI + inositol, using the HRSD as an assessment tool at baseline, and one, two, three, and four weeks. Second, there was no significant difference between the two treatment groups. Third, as with the above results, combined antidepressants show no evidence for additive effects, such as MAOI + TCA including CPZ (Figure 10) or TCA + lithium. Interestingly, by contrast, augmentation by lithium or MAOI after a failed course of antidepressant treatment was effective. Therefore, the study of the Levine group might be worth continuing with the combined medication methods of inositol + effective antidepressants to obtain more detailed knowledge [38, 80].

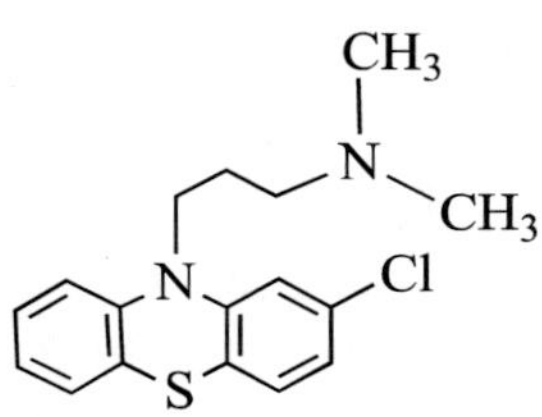

chlorpromazine (**22**)

Figure 10. Chlorpromazine (**22**).

2.1.2.5. Improvements in Depression Symptoms with Inositol

Losses of postmortem robust glial cells in the human PFC and more subtle neuronal changes were observed in MDD autopsy, and the glial marker inositol in MDD was subject to potential confounding from proton magnetic resonance spectroscopy (1H-MRS) of the MDD patients. In 2005 a group from the Department of Psychiatry, University of Alberta, Edmonton, Alberta, Canada examined whether administration of inositol can increase inositol levels in the prefrontal cortex/anterior cingulate cortex (PFC/ACC). 1H-MRS has been used as a noninvasive diagnostic method to measure the biochemical substances in the brain with AD and aMCI [81, 82].

Studies based on the diagnostic method for prediction of conversion from aMCI to AD used 13 nonmedicated moderate-severe MDD patients and 13 matched control subjects (six males and seven females). 1H-MRS stimulated echo acquisition mode spectra of nonmedicated moderate-severe MDD patients obtained from PFC/ACC. Their metabolite data from the echo acquisition mode spectra were adjusted for tissue composition. Second, MDD patients showed significantly lower inositol/creatine ratios (MI/Cr: ~0.94) compared to MI/Cr: ~1.32 of matched control subjects. The results suggest that reduction of inositol in PFC/ACC in MDD patients could be a consequence of glial loss or altered glial metabolism. Moreover, glial decrease measured from glial markers in vivo might help to support understanding of the pathophysiology of MDD [83].

2.1.2.6. Reduced Symptoms of Depression with Inositol

In 2007 a group from the Centre for Research in Neurodegenerative Diseases, University of Toronto, Ontario, Canada examined whether scyllo-inositol (Figure 11), one of the stereoisomers of inositol, has a sustained ability to treat TgCRND8 mice at advanced stages of AD-like pathology. As a result, first, the insoluble amyloid beta40 peptide (Abeta40), amyloid beta42 peptide (Abeta42), and plaque accumulation of amyloid beta deposited in the brain of scyllo-inositol treated TgCRND8 mice showed significantly greater decrease compared to a decrease of three insoluble proteins in untreated TgCRND8 mice. The size and growth of plaque accumulation in both Abeta40 and Abeta42 were inhibited by oral administration of scyllo-inositol.

Second, examining the effects of scyllo-inositol within the CNS, gas chromatography–mass spectrometry (GC-MS) was used to measure inositol and scyllo-inositol concentrations after oral administration. Additionally, it was examined how closely scyllo-inositol and inositol are interregulated in the CNS and whether scyllo-inositol, if elevated within the CNS would incorporate into phosphatidylinositol lipids. As a result, CSF levels of scyllo-inositol increased after oral administration of scyllo-inositol but not oral administration of inositol. Additionally, oral administration of scyllo-inositol caused increased levels of scyllo-inositol in the TgCRND8 mice brains. Moreover, scyllo-inositol, even at elevated levels, did not incorporate into the phosphatidylinositol family of lipids.

Results suggest that scyllo-inositol accumulates within the CNS up to 10 times endogenous levels, and increasing levels in TgCRND8 mice brains after oral administration of scyllo-inositol also protect progression of AD. On the other hand, oral administration of scyllo-inositol did not interfere with phosphatidylinositol lipid production [84].

2.1.2.7. Reduced Symptoms of Depression with Inositol

Toxicity of soluble amyloid-β (Aβ) is stronger compared to toxicity of fibrillar amyloid-β (fibrillar Aβ) in plaques [85, 86]. In 1995 a group from the Magnetic Resonance Spectroscopy Unit, Huntington Medical Research Institutes, Pasadena, CA examined distinctions between probable AD and other dementias (ODs) and normality in the elderly, with 244 subjects. There were 114 patients—65 AD patients, 39 OD patients, and 10 frontal lobe dementia patients (FLD patients)—plus 98 patients without dementia and 32 healthy control subjects. AD patients showed reduced levels of *N*-acetylaspartate (NAA) (Figure 12) and increased levels of inositol. OD patients showed significantly reduced levels of NAA but normal levels of inositol. On the MI/NAA ratio, AD patients could be easily distinguished from healthy control subjects, with 83% sensitivity and 98% specificity compared to the MI/NAA ratio of healthy control subjects. Additionally, with the MI/creatine ratio, OD patients were distinguished from AD patients and FLD patients with 80% negative predictive rate, 82% sensitivity, and 64% specificity.

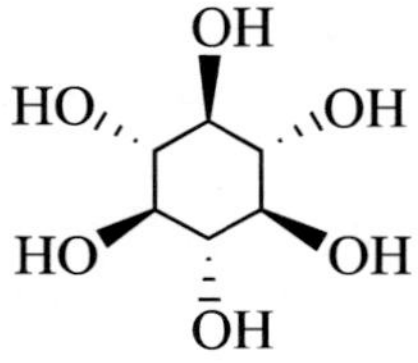

scyllo-inositol (**23**)

Figure 11. Scyllo-inositol (**23**).

These results suggest that 1H-MRS enables clinical identification of mild-moderate AD patients and diagnosis of probable AD patients using the specificity and sensitivity of 1H-MRS [87]. Minimal inhibition for formation or oligomerization of soluble Aβ may be effective for inhibition or prevention of AD progression and increase (worsening).

In 2010 a group from the A. A. Martinos Center for Biomedical Imaging, Department of Radiology, Massachusetts General Hospital and Harvard Medical School, examined whether low, therapeutically useful doses of scyllo-inositol lead to increases in scyllo-inositol in two brain regions (hippocampus and frontal cortex) and in two mouse models, AD mouse APP×PS1 and APP×PS1×tau mouse, plus a triple transgenic mouse model that harbors three mutant human genes—amyloid precursor protein (APPswe), presenilin-1 ($PS1_{M146V}$), and tau_{P301L}. Mice were scyllo-inositol fed and regular-diet fed. The ability was investigated to measure regionally specific drug increases in conjunction with therapeutic response.

First, on the effects of scyllo-inositol administration in the hippocampus and frontal cortex of triple transgene mice using high-resolution magic angle spinning (HR-MAS), the value of the scyllo-inositol/creatine ratio in the scyllo-inositol-fed mice showed ~0.074 (~2.38-fold increase) for the hippocampus compared to ~0.031 of regular-diet mice (control), and showed ~0.035 (2.18 times) for the frontal cortex compared to ~0.016 of the regular-diet mice (control), respectively.

However, the value of the inositol/creatine ratio in the scyllo-inositol fed mice was ~0.701 (~0.93-fold increase) for the hippocampus compared to ~0.748 of the regular-diet mice (control), and showed ~0.736 (~0.96 times) for the frontal cortex compared to ~0.759 of the regular-diet mice (control), respectively. Similarly, with 11 chemical/creatine ratios—GABA/creatine ratio, acetate/creatine ratio, alanine/creatine ratio, aspartate/creatine ratio, choline/creatine ratio, glutamate/creatine ratio, glutamine/creatine ratio, glycine/creatine ratio, lactate/creatine ratio, NAA/creatine ratio, and taurine/creatine ratio (Figure 12)—there were minor changes in the NMR spectra between scyllo-inositol fed mice and regular-diet mice (control) for the metabolites except scyllo-inositol/creatine. Glutamate and NAA values were higher in the frontal cortex than in the hippocampus for both the scyllo-inositol treated mice and the regular-diet mice. The scyllo-inositol/creatine values were smaller in both the regular-diet mice and the scyllo-inositol treated mice in the frontal cortex compared to the hippocampus. There was little overlap of scyllo-inositol values between the groups as a function of diet. Second, on the effects of scyllo-inositol treatment in the frontal cortex of APP×PS1 double transgenic mice using brain extracts, all the mice showed the brain extract spectra as follows:

Content (μmol/g tissue) of scyllo-inositol in the scyllo-inositol fed APPxPS1 triple transgene mice showed ~0.264 (~2.97-fold increase) for the frontal cortex compared to ~0.089 of the regular-diet mice (control). However, on the other 16 chemical contents, such as gamma-aminobutyric acid (GABA), acetate, alanine, aspartate, choline, creatine, glutamate, glutamine, glutathione (GSH), glycine, lactate, NAA, *N*-acetylaspartyl-glutamate (NAAG), succinate, taurine, and inositol in the mice frontal cortex, there were little changes in the nuclear magnetic resonance spectra (NMR spectra) between scyllo-inositol fed mice and regular diet mice (control) for any of the metabolites except scyllo-inositol. There was no overlap of scyllo-inositol values for the frontal cortex between the groups as a function of diet. The content (μmol/g tissue) in the frontal cortex for the scyllo-inositol fed mice group was the lowest 0.214 for NAAG and the highest 8.952 for taurine, respectively. The content (μmol/g tissue) in the frontal cortex for the regular diet mice group was the lowest, 0.089, for scyllo-inositol, and the highest, 9.014, for taurine, respectively.

From the above results, these mice were treated with water containing scyllo-inositol at a concentration of 16.5 mg/L. This consumption is equivalent to a dose of ~3.3 mg/kg/day. It suggests that such a high dose, 2,000-4,000 mg/day, will likely not lead to much higher intracerebral levels of scyllo-inositol compared to the intracerebral level that can be attained using lower doses (250 mg/day) of scyllo-inositol. Additionally, it is expected that high-resolution magic angle spinning (HR-MAS) might prove one of the invaluable methods in determining the minimum effective dose (MED) of scyllo-inositol treatment for AD patients [88].

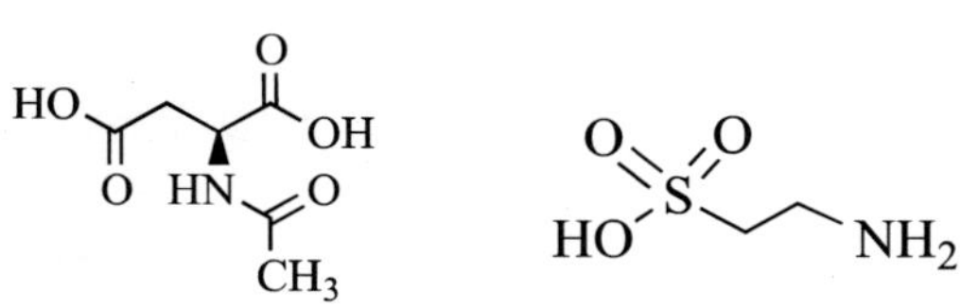

N-acetylaspartate (NAA. **24**)

taurine (**25**)

Figure 12. *N*-Acetylaspartate (NAA. **24**) and taurine (**25**)

2.1.3. Folic Acid and Folinic Acid

2.1.3.1. Folic Acid Deficiency during Early Neurodevelopment Predisposed to Schizophrenia

In 1996 a group from the Department of Psychiatry, Columbia University tried to confirm the hypothesis from previous studies that early prenatal nutritional deficiency is associated with an increased risk for schizophrenia [89-91]. Regarding the method of birth cohorts, the risk for schizophrenia was compared by using exposed and unexposed persons of early gestation during the Dutch Hunger Winter of 1944/1945 on birth cohorts in six cities with populations larger than 40,000, such as Amsterdam, the Hague, Haarlem, Leiden, Rotterdam, and Utrecht in western Netherlands during 1944 through 1946. The frequency of schizophrenia inpatients at ages 24-48 years in the exposed and unexposed birth cohorts was ascertained from a national psychiatric registry.

Regarding schizophrenia in birth cohorts exposed and unexposed to early prenatal nutritional deficiency during the Dutch Hunger Winter of 1944 through 1945, cumulative incidence /1,000 persons and relative risk (RR) for all persons was 3.8 and 2.0 for the exposed birth cohort of October 15 through December 31, 1945 (EX2 cohort), 2.0 and 1.1 for the exposed birth cohort of August 1 through October 14, 1945 (EX1 cohort), and 1.9 for the unexposed birth cohort of August 1 through October 14, 1945, respectively. Cumulative incidence /1,000 persons and RR for men was 4.1 and 1.9 for the EX2 cohort, 2.5 and 1.2 for the EX1 cohort, and 2.2 for the unexposed cohort, respectively. Cumulative incidence /1,000 persons and RR for women was 3.5 and 2.2 for the EX2 cohort, 1.5 and 0.9 for the EX1 cohort, and 1.6 for the unexposed cohort, respectively (original Table 2). Results show risk (cumulative incidence /1,000 persons for schizophrenia of the EX2 cohort was significantly higher compared to the risk of the unexposed cohort. RR did not show a big difference in gender of men and women. RR of the onset of schizophrenia in the EX2 cohort of both men and women was higher compared to RR of the EX1 cohort of both men and women.

Second, on risk for 17 successive birth cohorts of January-February 1944 to November-December 1946, risk (cumulative incidence/1,000 persons for schizophrenia showed the highest ~3.8 in the EX2 cohort, and the risk of 16 other birth cohorts was ~1.2-2.1.

Third, on congenital neural defects in males of birth cohorts exposed and unexposed to early prenatal nutritional deficiency during the Dutch Hunger Winter of 1944 through 1945 (prevalence data), the cumulative incidence/

1,000 persons and RR for all persons was 3.9 and 2.5 for the EX2 cohort, 1.7 and 1.1 for the EX1 cohort, and 1.5 and for the unexposed cohort, respectively. From the results, the EX2 cohort showed a significant excess (RR value: 2.5) of congenital neurodefects. On the other hand, the EX1 cohort showed no significant excess (RR value: 1.1).

Fourth, regarding the incidence data under the narrow and broad definitions of schizophrenia in birth cohorts exposed and unexposed to early prenatal nutritional deficiency during the Dutch Hunger Winter of 1944/1945, first, on the narrow definition of schizophrenia, the cumulative incidence/1,000 persons of the most recent discharged patients was 3.8 for the EX2 cohort and 1.9 for the unexposed cohort, and the RR (EX2 cohort vs. unexposed cohort) was 2.0.

Cumulative incidence/1,000 persons of any discharged patients was 4.5 for the EX2 cohort and 2.4 for the unexposed cohort, and the RR (EX2 cohort vs. unexposed cohort) was 1.9. Cumulative incidence/1,000 persons of any discharged or admission patients was 4.8 for the EX2 cohort and 2.8 for the unexposed cohort, and RR (EX2 cohort vs. unexposed cohort) was 1.7.

Second, regarding the broad definition of schizophrenia, cumulative incidence/1,000 persons of the most recent discharged patients was 5.3 for the EX2 cohort and 3.6 for the unexposed cohort, and RR (EX2 cohort vs. unexposed cohort) was 1.5.

Cumulative incidence/1,000 persons of any discharged patients was 6.0 for the EX2 cohort and 3.7 for the unexposed cohort, and RR (EX2 cohort vs. unexposed cohort) was 1.6. Cumulative incidence/1,000 persons of any discharged or admission patients was 6.4 for the EX2 cohort and 4.3 for the unexposed cohort, and RR (EX2 cohort vs. unexposed cohort) was 1.5.

Fifth, regarding incidence among the EX2 cohort vs. all other cohorts born 1944 through 1946 of schizophrenia in birth cohorts of nonfamine cities within the Netherlands, cumulative incidence/1,000 persons under the narrow definition of schizophrenia was 1.6 for the EX2 cohort and 1.4 for all other cohorts, and the RR (EX2 cohort vs. all other cohorts) was 1.1.

The current study used group data to define actual individuals such as the exposed birth cohort of October 15 through December 31, 1945 (EX2 cohort) and the exposed birth cohorts of August 1 through October 14, 1945 (EX1 cohort).

Unconfounded estimates on the deficiencies of particular nutrients cannot be determined from the available data. Caloric deficiency, protein deficiency, and deficiencies of specific micronutrients occurred simultaneously during the Dutch Hunger Winter, and each of these deficiencies affected brain development in animal tests [92, 93]. To obtain individual exposure data and specify relevant exposure, the research group is presently conducting a study of the large birth cohorts in the U.S., and stored prenatal material serum samples are available to measure the prenatal nutritional exposures for schizophrenic patients and the matched controls of prenatal nutritional unexposures (normal nutrition intake cohorts).

Third, because the time of birth could not be known, the time of conception must be inferred. Therefore, conception time must be estimated at maturity pregnancy. The great majority of births including schizophrenic births and birth after prenatal famine exposure were observed at full term [94, 95]. However, if short gestations were more frequent among schizopherenic births compared to other births, the effect of the misclassification could deflate estimates of the true RR for the EX2 cohort.

Fourth, complete data on congenital neural defects were available only for male congenital neuropathy patient from their recruitment inspection. On the other hand, the morbidity data from recruitment inspection, the basis for a priori specification regarding timing of exposure, were lacking for female congenital neuropathy patients.

Fifth, data on social class of origin were not available. There was no relationship between schizophrenia and low social class of origin [96]. Because incidence of schizophrenia for the EX2 birth cohort was weighed toward the upper classes, any such association would tend to reduce the estimated RR in the present study.

These discussions suggest that prenatal nutritional deficiency may be one of the origins of risk for schizophrenia in some cases. This idea may be strongly supported by these facts which the incidence of neural tube defects can be reduced substantially by nutritional supplementation in early pregnancy [97, 98, 99, 100].

2.1.3.2. Folic Acid and Folinic Acid

In 2002 a group from the Depression Clinical and Research Program, Department of Psychiatry, Massachusetts General Hospital assessed the efficacy of methylfolate (Figure 13) as an adjunctive treatment among adults with MDD and inadequate response to an SSRI.

First, 22 SSRI-refractory depression patients (9 males and 13 females; average age 45.2 years) who satisfied one of three conditions were enrolled in this eight-week prospective open trial. The MDD patients had partial or no response to an SSRI after at least four weeks of treatment, and 17-item Hamilton Depression Rating Scale (HAM-D-17) score of >12.

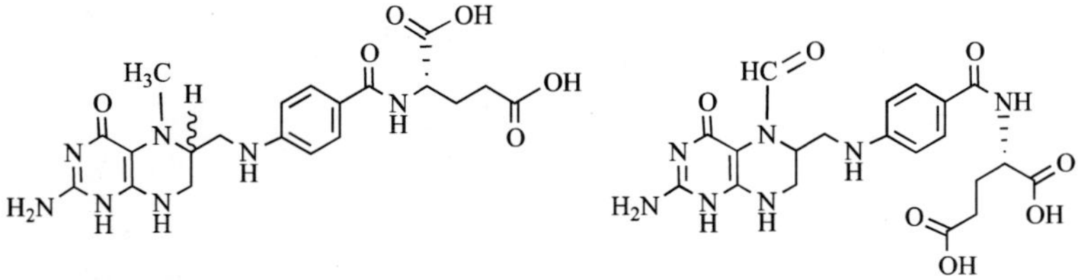

methylfolate (levomefolic acid.. **26**) folinic acid (leucovorin. **27**)

Figure 13. Methylfolate (levomefolic acid. **26**) and folinic acid (leucovorin. **27**).

Second, according to the exclusion criteria in this study, SSRI-refractory depression patients now using anticonvulsants or psychotropics other than an SSRI or with B12 deficiency have been excluded. Folinic acid (Figure 13) at 15-30 mg/day, metabolized to methylfolate, was added in combined administration with SSRIs to the 22 SSRI-refractory depression patients. First, methylfolate levels in the serum in SSRI-refractory depression patients increased significantly from 28 ± 19 ng/mL to 301 ± 203 ng/mL. Second, HAM-D-17 scores among 31% of SSRI-refractory depression patients decreased from 19.1 ± 3.9 to 12.8 ± 7.0. However, 27% of the intent-to-treat (ITT) SSRI-refractory depression patients showed the response, representing 50% or more reduction on HAM-D-17 scores, and only 19% of SSRI-refractory depression patients and 18% of ITT SSRI-refractory depression patients showed remission with HAM-D-17 score <7. These results suggest that folinic acid appears to be modestly effective as an adjunct among SSRI-refractory depressed individuals with normal methylfolate levels [101].

In 2000 a group from the MRC Neuropsychiatry Laboratory, West Park Hospital, Surrey, Epsom, UK examined whether coadministration of folic acid (Figure 14) would enhance the antidepressant action of fluoxetine. Patients were randomised to receive a capsule of either 500 μg folic acid or an identical-looking placebo capsule to take with 20 mg fluoxetine daily for 10 weeks. Among 127 patients eligible after the 10-week trial, 51 of 62 patients randomly assigned folic acid completed the trial and 58 of 65 patients randomly assigned to placebo completed the trial.

First, regarding the comparison on content (ng/mL) of the plasma folate at baseline and Week 10, women were 4.04 at baseline and 12.70 at Week 10 for patients who had received fluoxetine plus 500 μg folic acid, and 4.28 at baseline and 4.27 at Week 10 for patients who had received fluoxetine plus placebo, respectively. Men were 4.58 at baseline and 8.70 at Week 10 for patients who had received fluoxetine plus 500 μg folic acid and 4.18 at baseline and 4.01 at Week 10 for patients who had received fluoxetine plus placebo, respectively. From the results, both male and female patients receiving fluoxetine plus folic acid showed a significantly better response at Week 10 compared to response of patients who had received fluoxetine plus placebo.

Second, regarding the comparison on content (μmol/L) of the plasma homocysteine (Figure 14) at baseline and Week 10, women were 9.46 at baseline and 7.51 at Week 10 for patients who had received fluoxetine plus 500 μg folic acid, and 8.56 at baseline and 9.36 at Week 10 for patients who had received fluoxetine plus placebo, respectively. Men were 9.65 at baseline and 9.01 at Week 10 for patients who had received fluoxetine plus 500 μg folic acid, and 9.92 at baseline and 10.21 at Week 10 for patients who had received fluoxetine plus placebo, respectively. From the results, female patients receiving fluoxetine plus folic acid showed a significant decrease at Week 10 compared to response of patients who had received fluoxetine plus placebo. However, the decrease was less in men compared to the decrease in women.

Third, regarding the comparison on content (pg/mL) of the plasma vitamin B12 (Figure 15) at baseline and Week 10, women were 317.4 at baseline and 322.8 at Week 10 for patients who had received fluoxetine plus 500 μg folic acid, and 378.0 at baseline and 377.3 at Week 10 for patients who had received fluoxetine plus placebo, respectively. Men were 315.9 at baseline and 285.2 at Week 10 for patients who had received fluoxetine plus 500 μg folic acid, and 396.0 at baseline and 405.8 at Week 10 for patients who had received fluoxetine plus placebo, respectively. From the results, both male and female patients receiving fluoxetine plus folic acid did not show a significant difference at Week 10 compared to response of patients who had received fluoxetine plus placebo.

Fourth, on the comparison of ITT analysis, HRSD scores at baseline and Week 10, women were 27.0 at baseline and 6.8 at Week 10 for patients who had received fluoxetine plus 500 μg folic acid, and 26.7 at baseline and 11.4 at Week 10 for patients who had received fluoxetine plus placebo, respectively. Men were 26.6 at baseline and 10.9 at Week 10 for patients who had received fluoxetine plus 500 μg folic acid, and 26.4 at baseline and 9.7 at Week 10 for patients who had received fluoxetine plus placebo, respectively. From the results, patients receiving fluoxetine plus folic acid had a significantly better response at Week 10 compared to that of patients who had received fluoxetine plus placebo.

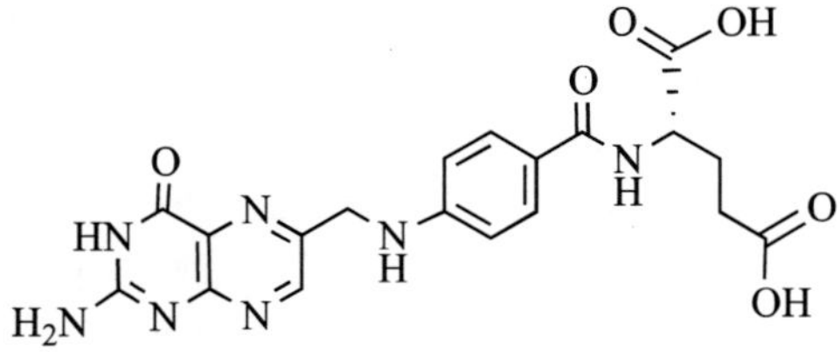

folic acid (folate. **28**)

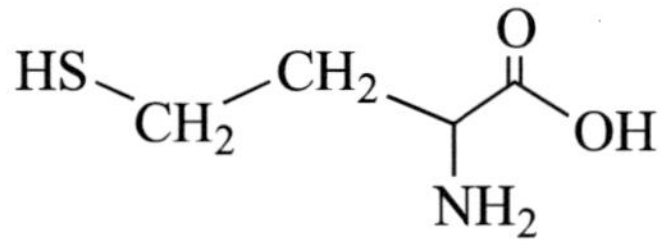

homocysteine (**29**)

Figure 14. Folic acid (folate. **28**) and homocysteine (**29**).

Fifth, on the recovered patients vs. the patients who did not recover (the remainder) according to HRS score of 9 at completion, women were 24 (72.7%) for recovered patients ($\leqq$9) and 9 (27.3%) for the remainder (>9) on patients who had received fluoxetine plus 500 μg folic acid, and 17 (47.2%) for recovered patients ($\leqq$9) and 19 (52.8%) for the remainder (>9) on patients who had received fluoxetine plus placebo, respectively. Men were 9 (50.0%) for recovered patients ($\leqq$9) and 9 (50.0%) for the remainder (>9) on patients who had received fluoxetine plus 500 μg folic acid, and 11 (50.0%) for recovered patients ($\leqq$9) and 11 (50.0%) for the remainder (>9) on patients who had received fluoxetine plus placebo, respectively. From the results, 72.7% (HRS score of 9) of women patients who had received fluoxetine plus 500 μg folic acid showed a more significant recovery rate compared to HRS 9: 47.2% in women patients (remainders) who had received fluoxetine plus placebo.

From the above results (First to Fifth), it suggests that, especially, the application to females of folic acid for enhancing the antidepressant action of fluoxetine or other SSRIs is clinically one of the beneficial treatments for the development and substantial effect in the treatment of serious depression. On the other hand, antidepressant action of SSRIs with folic acid for men patients in this study showed less antidepressant action compared to antidepressant action of female patients [102].

2.1.3.3. Folic Acid Deficiency during Early Neurodevelopment Predisposed to Schizophrenia

In 2005 a group from the Bio-X Center, Shanghai Jiao Tong University, Shanghai determined whether those who endured a massive 1959-1961 famine in China experienced similar results of schizophrenia. On the evidence of famine from birth rates and mortality rates, population and birth, death, and growth rate/1,000 individuals living in Wuhu, China and its six surrounding counties before, during, and after the famine years 1959-1961 are as follows. Vital statistics of population (VSP) in 1957 was 1,699,779 for population, 41.21 for birth rate, 10.27 for death rate, and 30.94 for growth rate. VSP in 1958 was 1,767,835 for population, 28.28 for birth rate, 17.77 for death rate, and 10.51 for growth rate. VSP in 1959 was 1,691,266 for population, 20.92 for birth rate, 32.13 for death rate and -11.16 for growth rate. VSP in 1960 was 1,501,444 for population, 8.61 for birth rate, 92.61 for death rate, and -84.00 for growth rate. VSP in 1961 was 1,454,320 for population, 11.06 for birth rate, 15.63 for death rate, and -4.57 for growth rate. And VSP in 1962 was 1,536,282 for population, 50.4 for birth rate, 10.95 for death rate, and 39.45 for growth rate. From the results, birth rates showed significant decrease by ~80% for the years 1960 and 1961. Mortality started rising in 1959 (-11.16) and peaked in 1960 (-84.00). Overall mortality rate in Anhui was 12%; however, overall mortality for Wuhu and its surrounding six counties was 15%. This suggests that VSP provides conclusive evidence of famine in Wuhu in the years 1959-1961.

Second, on the increased risk of schizophrenia, the clinicodemographic information on schizophrenia cases born before, during, and after the famine years was as follows. The decline in birth rates during the famine years 1959-1961 was accompanied by a decline in the absolute number for schizophrenia onset in people born during the famine years 1959-1961. However, as a proportion of total births in each year (1957-1962), the cumulative risk of schizophrenia during 1960 and 1961 increased significantly compared to schizophrenia onset rates before or after.

Third, on the numbers of cases of schizophrenia born in each of the years 1956 to 1965 in Wuhu and surrounding counties, increased risk was similar in hospitalized and nonhospitalized cases. Both sexes were equally affected, and there was no difference in age of schizophrenia onset among those born before, during, or after the famine years.

Mortality-adjusted risks were calculated using estimates of cumulative mortality rates derived from the 1982 and the 1988 population surveys. Both population surveys of 1982 and 1988 showed cumulative mortality rates of 35%-40% among children conceived or born during the famine years 1959-1961 and cumulative mortality rates of 20%-30% among children born in the famine years 1959-1961 immediately preceding the famine. For persons born in 1963 and after, cumulative mortality rates decreased to 5%-10%.

Comparing famine and aftermath between the famine years 1959-1961 and years (1956-1958 and 1963-1965) well away from the famine to produce

RR, mortality-adjusted RR was 2.3 (95% confidence interval, 1.99-2.65) for those born in 1960 and 1.93 (95% confidence interval, 1.68-2.23) for those born in 1961, respectively.

These results suggest that prenatal exposure to famine increases risk of schizophrenia in later life. Surprisingly, the findings in this study are internally consistent and reproduce almost exactly the Dutch famine of 1944–45. Because the Chinese and Dutch are different populations in ethnic and cultural observations, it suggests that the results obtained by this experiment can be strongly adapted in all ethnicities of the world under famine, showing that prenatal exposure to famine increases risk of schizophrenia in later life [103].

2.1.3.4. Improvement in Schizophrenia with Combined Administration of Folic Acid and Vitamin 12

Schizophrenia is a chronic psychiatric illness separated into three categories: positive symptoms of schizophrenia: delusions, hallucinations, and disorganization or demolition symptoms; negative symptoms of schizophrenia: apathy, social withdrawal, and loss of emotional expressiveness; and cognitive impairment (cognitive deficits).

Antipsychotic medications control positive symptoms to allow most patients to live safely within the community. On the other hand, negative symptoms of schizophrenia and cognitive deficits have many obstacles for which effective treatment is not yet known [104].

Next-generation sequencing (NGS) methods exist for genome-wide genetic marker development and genotyping using restriction enzyme digestion of target genomes to reduce complexity of the target. NGS methods include reduced-representation sequencing using reduced-representation libraries (RRLs) or complexity reduction of polymorphic sequences (CRoPS), restriction-site-associated DNA sequencing (RAD-seq), and low coverage genotyping [105].

In 2010 a group from the Department of Psychiatry and Neuropsychology, EURON, Maastricht University Medical Centre, the Netherlands reviewed a complex and heterogeneous genetic vulnerability to schizophrenia that interacts with environmental factors using NGS methods.

First, the common polymorphisms robustly associated with schizophrenia have been identified as Zinc finger protein 804A (ZNF804A) of a protein encoded by the ZNF804A gene in humans, transcription factor 4 (TCF-4) of immunoglobulin transcription factor 2 (ITF-2), major histocompatibility complex (MHC), and neurogranin of a calmodulin-binding protein that facilitates long-term potentiation by NGS methods.

ZNF804A is expressed broadly throughout the brain, especially in the developing hippocampus and the cortex, as well as in the adult cerebellum [106]. TCF-4 is especially a protein encoded by the TCF4 gene which related to Pitt-Hopkins Syndrome in humans [107, 108].

Major histocompatibility complex (MHC) is a set of cell surface proteins essential for the acquired immune system to recognize foreign molecules in vertebrates, which in turn determines histocompatibility. Schizophrenia's strongest genetic association at a population level involves the variation in the MHC locus [109].

On the action of neurogranin, increasing plasticity in neurons of the PFC has been proposed as a possible therapeutic tool to reduce extinction for neuropathies such as posttraumatic stress disorder (PTSD), schizophrenia, and addiction. Neurogranin overexpression in PFC enhanced long-term potentiation and increased rates of extinction learning of both fear conditioning and sucrose self-administration. It suggests that the elevated neurogranin function within the PFC can enhance local plasticity and increase the rate of extinction learning across different behavioral tasks, meaning neurogranin can provide a molecular link between enhanced plasticity and enhanced extinction for the neuropathies [110].

Second, in addition to ZNF804A, TCF-4, MHC, and neurogranin from the above described components, the copy-number variants (CNVs) by chromosomal changes of six hotspots, 1q21.1, 2p16.3, 15q11.2, 15q13.3, 16p11.2, and 22q11.2 microduplications were convincingly related to schizophrenia risk. These studies suggest considerable genetic overlap with bipolar disorders, in particular common polymorphisms and neuro-developmental disorders such as autism of CNVs [111].

Third, etiological models of psychosis are needed, integrating genetic risk with environmental factors. For example, amyloid beta protein and the speckled structure formed in cells under the environmental impact on gene expression. Epigenetics deals with change of gene function not in DNA sequence but when transmitted through cell division due to methylation, etc. Convergence of genes and environment on common biological pathways brings about larger antischizophrenia effects by gene-environment interaction, compared to antischizophrenia effects of genes themselves in human or genes in an isolated environment without gene-environment interaction [112].

In 2013 a group from the Department of Psychiatry, Massachusetts General Hospital studied whether folic acid plus vitamin B12 (Figure 15) supplementation reduces negative symptoms of schizophrenia and whether functional variants in folate-related genes influence the therapeutic response.

In the primary study, adjunctive folate and vitamin B12 supplementation was effective for positive and negative symptoms of schizophrenia with a methylenetetrahydrofolate reductase deficiency (MTHFRD) genotype of MTHFR 677C > T genotype [113].

Also examined was whether folate and vitamin B12 supplementation could selectively improve negative symptoms, according to the scale for assessment of negative symptoms (SANS), a rating scale measuring negative symptoms in schizophrenia. This SANS pattern for negative symptoms would be applied by MTHFR defective genotype. Post hoc analyses were done of relevant subscales and relationships in RBC folate levels between genotype and baseline as well as changes in folate levels over time.

First, among 189 patients screened, 140 eligible patients were at random administered either the supplementation with 2 mg folate/day and 400 μg vitamin B12 /day for 94 patients, or the supplementation of matching placebo for 46 patients. A total of 121 patients (86%) completed 16 weeks of treatment.

On change with time in level (ng/mL) of RBC folate, first, levels (ng/mL) in the placebo group were ~440 at baseline, ~480 at Week 8, and ~460 at Week 16. Levels (ng/mL) in the active group (treated group) were ~460 at baseline, ~550 at Week 8, and ~570 at Week 16. The active groups showed higher levels (ng/mL) of RBC folate over time, yielding significant between-group differences compared to RBC levels of the placebo groups.

Regarding levels (ng/mL) of RBC folate in patients receiving active treatment among those grouped by a variant folate hydrolase 1 (FOLH1) 484T > C genotype, levels (ng/mL) of RBC folic acid for FOLH1 484T/T carrier patients was ~480 at baseline, ~560 at Week 8, and ~550 at Week 16. Levels (ng/mL) of RBC folate for FOLH1 484C/C carrier patients was ~300 at baseline, ~480 at Week 8, and ~590 at Week 16.

Regarding symptom change, first, before administration of two active components such as folate and vitamin B12 to patients with genotypes on the ITT analysis, the score (mean value with 95% confidence interval) of SANS was -0.19 for active group, 0.02 for placebo group, and -0.21 for difference between two groups, respectively. The PANSS positive score (mean value with 95% confidence interval) and PANSS total score of positive and negative syndrome scale (PANSS) was -0.06 and -0.21 for the active group, -0.04 and -0.22 for the placebo group, and -0.02 and 0.02 for the difference between the two groups, respectively. The score (mean value with 95% confidence interval) of Calgary depression rating scale (CDRS) was -0.02 for the active group, 0.04 for the placebo group, and -0.06 for the difference between the two groups, respectively.

After administration of two active components such as folic acid and vitamin B12 to patients with genotypes on the ITT analysis, the SANS score (mean value with 95% confidence interval) was -0.17 for the active group, 0.16 for the placebo group, and -0.33 for the difference between the two groups, respectively. The PANSS positive score (mean value with 95% confidence interval) and PANSS total score was -0.08 and -0.21 for the active group, -0.01 and -0.10 for the placebo group, and -0.06 and -0.11 for the difference between the two groups, respectively. The CDRS score (mean value with 95% confidence interval) was 0.004 for the active group, 0.35 for the placebo group, and 0.39 for the difference between the two groups, respectively. From the results, the active group (patients) who received folic acid and vitamin B12 showed significantly greater decrease in negative symptoms (-0.19 change in SANS score/week; 95% confidence interval, -0.35 to -0.03) compared to change in the placebo group. The same pattern also was evident for PANSS positive scores. For PANSS total score, both the active group and the placebo group improved significantly over time.

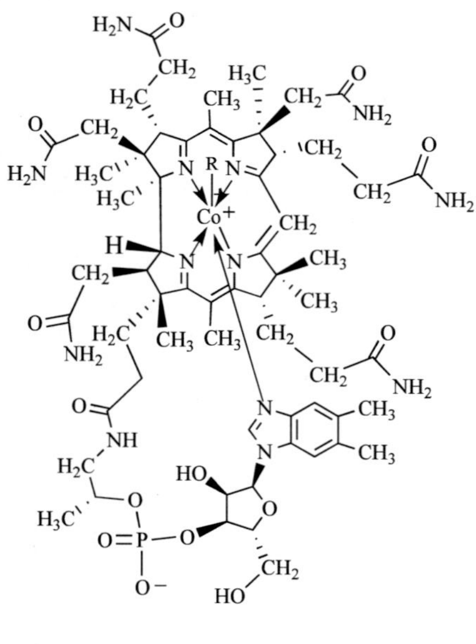

vitamin B12 (**30**) (R: 5'-deoxyadenosyl, Me, OH, CN)

Figure 15. Vitamin B12 (**30**).

Change from baseline of negative symptoms (SANS total score) among FOLH1 484T/T carrier patients and FOLH1 484C/C carrier patients: time-dependent change for FOLH1 484T/T carrier patients showed the more noticeable difference in active groups who received active treatment compared to time-dependent change of the placebo group. Second, the time-dependent change for FOLH1 484C/C carrier patients showed no noticeable difference in active groups who received active treatment compared to time-dependent change of the placebo group.

(First – Fourth) folate and vitamin B12 supplementation showed no clear effect for positive symptoms or depression scores, regardless of different genotypes such as FOLH1 484T/T or FOLH1 484C/C. This suggests that individual differences in folate metabolism related to the presence of common functional genetic variants has a bearing on treatment outcomes in disorders such as juvenile cerebral infarction, as well as negative symptoms of schizophrenia [114].

2.1.4. Herbs

In 2001 a group from the Department of Health Care Policy and the Center for Alternative Medicine Research and Education, Beth Israel Deaconess Medical Center, Harvard Medical School examined statistically the use of complementary therapy and alternative therapy to treat anxiety and depression by enhancing or speeding the response to antidepressants among depressed patients with mood disorder and anxiety disorders in the U.S.

To obtain information on the use of 24 CAMs for treatment of specific chronic conditions such as anxiety and depression, the epidemiological study was begun by using replies to questionnaires from 2,055 respondents with respondent ages 18 or older.

The four therapy types used were (1) cognitive feedback: relaxation techniques, imagery, self-help groups for mental health, hypnosis, biofeedback; (2) oral medication: herbal medicine, megavitamins, homeopathy, naturopathy; (3) physical treatment: massage, chiropractic, osteopathy, acupuncture, yoga; and (4) other therapies: spiritual healing by others, dietary modifications, lifestyle diet, special diet for losing or gaining weight, energy healing, aromatherapy, laughter, other therapy to treat pain, other lifestyle intervention program, folk remedies. Results suggest that the majority of people in the U.S. with self-defined anxiety attacks or severe depression have used complementary therapies and alternative therapies for treatment against these cognitive conditions. This means that dementia patients with these cognitive conditions are considerably more likely to use complementary therapies and alternative therapies compared to conventional medical treatments or mental health treatments.

Among these CAMs, oral medications, especially dietary supplements, show evidence in treatment of depression and, to a lesser extent, anxiety. *Hypericum perforatum* (St. John's wort) has been evaluated for treatment of depression. Two meta-analyses [115, 116] concluded that St. John's wort is better compared to placebo used in conventional pharmacotherapy for treatment of various depression severities [117].

2.1.5. SAMe

2.1.5.1. SAMe Cycle

SAMe (Figure 16) is a common cosubstrate involved in methyl group transfers, *trans*-sulfuration, and aminopropylation. Although these anabolic reactions occur throughout the body, most SAMe is produced and consumed in the liver [118].

Reactions that produce, consume, and regenerate SAMe. make up the SAM-e cycle. The SAM-e cycle is classified into three reactions: methylation (including DNA, proteins, phospholipids, neurotransmitters); *trans*-sulfuration (including cystathionine, cysteine, glutathione); and amino-propylation (including decarboxylated SAMe, MTA, and methionine) (Figure 16) [119].

2.1.5.2. Methionine Rich Nuts, Vegetables, and Fruits

Content (mg/100 g edible parts) of methionine-rich nuts, vegetables, and fruits are mainly as follows: Brazil nuts: 1,124; seeds, sesame seeds, whole, dried: 586; soybeans, mature seeds, dry roasted: 534; nuts, cashew nuts, raw: 362; seeds, sunflower seed kernels, dried: 494; peanuts, all types, dry roasted, without salt: 291; nuts, pine nuts, dried: 259; peanuts, all types, raw: 259; nuts, almonds, dry roasted, without salt added: 155; beans, white, mature seeds, cooked, boiled, without salt: 146; soybean, sprouts (soybeans, mature seeds, sprouted, raw): 138; nuts, chestnuts, Chinese, raw: 101; peas, green, raw: 82; maize (corn): 67 (corn, sweet, yellow, raw) and 67 (corn, sweet, white, raw); broadbeans (fava beans), mature seeds, raw: 213; nuts, chestnuts, Japanese, raw: 54; spinach, raw: 53; broccoli, raw: 38; garlic, raw: 76 [14]; leaf mustard, stems and leaves, raw: 38 [120]; potatoes, flesh and skin, raw: 32; asparagus, raw: 31; bamboo shoots, raw: 30; sweet potato, raw, unprepared: 24; kiwifruit, green, raw: 24; cauliflower, raw: 20 (cauliflower, raw) and 42 (cauliflower, green, raw); okra, raw: 21; lettuce, raw: 16 (lettuce, green leaf, raw) and 16 (lettuce, red leaf, raw); strawberry, raw fruit: 12; bananas, raw: 8 [14].

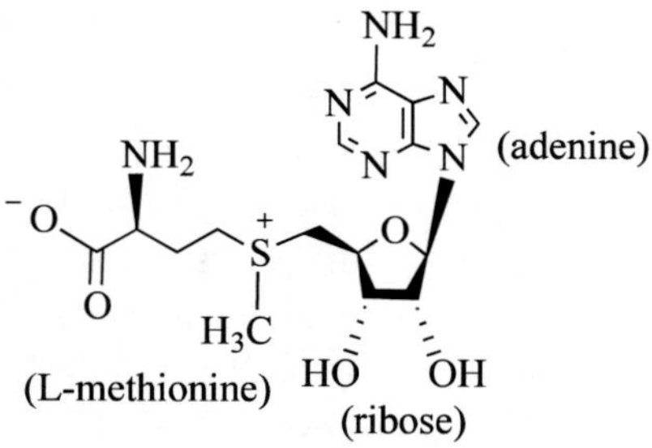

S-adenosyl-L-methionine (SAMe, **31**)

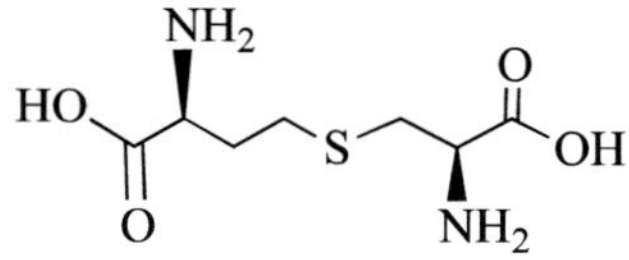

cystathionine (**32**)

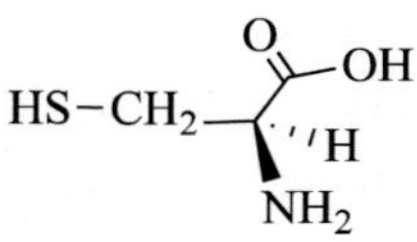

L-cysteine (**33**)

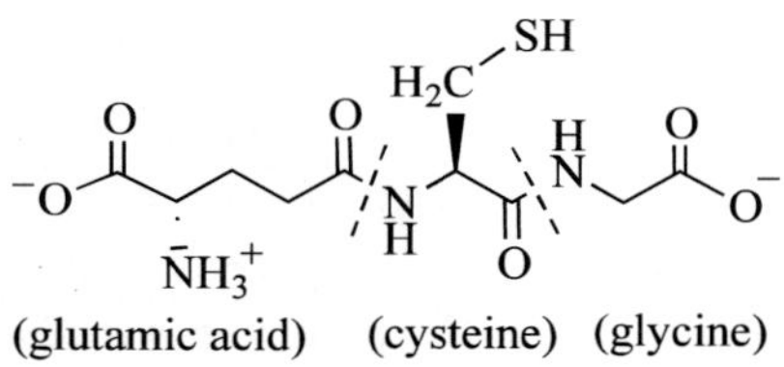

glutathione (GSH. gamma-L-Glu-L-Cys-Gly. **34**)

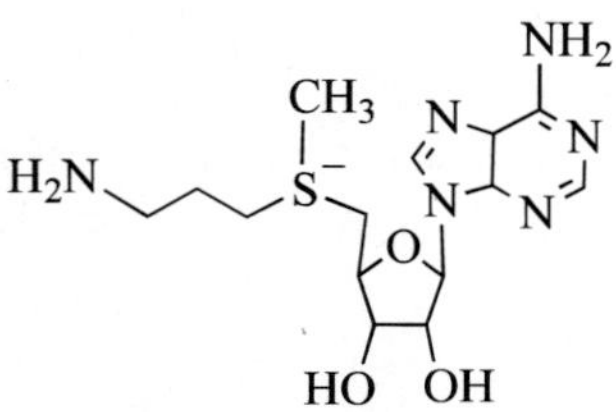

decarboxylated SAMe (deca-SAMe. decarboxylated *S*-adenosylmethionine (**35**)

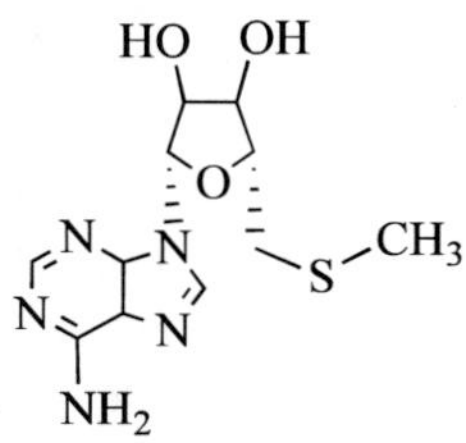

methyl-thioadenosine (MTA. **36**)

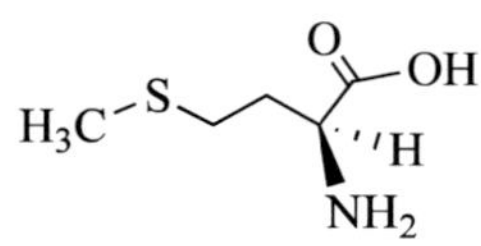

methionine (**37**)

Figure 16. *S*-Adenosyl-L-methionine (SAMe, **31**), cysathionine (**32**), L-cysteine (**33**), glutathione (GSH. gamma-L-Glu-L-Cys-Gly. **34**), decarboxylated SAMe (deca-SAMe. decarboxylated *S*-adenosylmethionine (**35**), methyl-thioadenosine (MTA. **36**) and methionine (**37**).

2.1.5.3. Clinical Meta-Analysis on SAMe

In 1994, Dr. Bressa of the Department of Psychiatry, University Cattolica Sacro Cuore School of Medicine, Rome, Italy examined by clinical meta-analysis SAMe antidepressant effect with a naturally occurring substance that is a major source of methyl groups in the brain. The meta-analysis assessed the effect of SAMe in treatment of depression by comparison with the effects of placebo and standard tricyclic antidepressants such as CPZ. SAMe showed a greater response rate compared to response rate of placebo, representing a global effect size ranging from 17% to 38%, based on the response definition. Additionally, SAMe showed an antidepressant effect comparable with that of standard tricyclic antidepressants. The results indicate that antidepressant effect of SAMe in treatment of depressive syndromes and disorders is superior to the effect of placebo and comparable to the effect of standard tricyclic antidepressants. The study suggests that SAMe as a naturally occurring compound has relatively few side effects; SAMe is becoming one of the adjuvant therapies for depression [121].

2.1.5.4. Safety, Tolerability, and Efficacy of SAMe

In 2004 a group from the Depression Clinical and Research Program, Massachusetts General Hospital, Department of Psychiatry, Harvard Medical School evaluated the safety, tolerability, and efficacy of oral *S*-adenosyl-L-methionine tosylate (Figure 17). For partial responders and nonresponders, it is adjunct to venlafaxine (Figure 17), a serotonin-norepinephrine reuptake inhibitor (SNRI) antidepressant. Antidepressant-treated adult outpatients (23 or 30) with persisting MDD received 800-1,600 mg of SAMe-tosylate over a six-week trial. At the same time, the patients were required to be on a stable (≥4 weeks), minimally adequate dose of an SSRI or venlafaxine (fluoxetine/paroxetine/citalopram ≥20 mg/day, escitalopram ≥10 mg/day, sertraline ≥50 mg/day, or venlafaxine ≥75 mg/day) (Figure 17). Additionally, all patients needed to meet *DSM 4th ed.* criteria for current major depressive disorder and have a 17-item Hamilton depression scale (HAM-D17) score ≥14 at screening and baseline visits.

First, regarding the change of scores on HAM-D17 on 30 antidepressant-treated adult outpatients by ITT analysis, the questionnaire scores of the patients were ~17.8 at baseline (Week 0), ~13.1 at Week 1, ~13.1 at Week 2, ~10.8 at Week 3, ~11.0 at Week 4, and ~10.0 at Week 6.

Subsequently, regarding the change of scores on the HAM-D17 of 23 antidepressant-treated adult outpatients, questionnaire scores were ~17.8 at baseline (Week 0), ~12.9 at Week 1, ~13.0 at Week 2, ~10.4 at Week 3, ~10.5 at Week 4, and ~9.2 at Week 6. Results show a significant decrease in patient depression severity, with significant high score differences between baseline (at Week 0) and endpoint (Week 6) by the HAM-D–17 in both ITT and completer patient groups.

Second, significant improvements in both the symptom questionnaire (SQ)-depression scores and SQ-anxiety scores were observed statistically between the baseline (Week 0) and the endpoint (Week 6), but the improvement in SQ-anger/hostility scores could not be observed in ITT and completer patient groups. Third, improvements in SQ-somatic symptom scores, or SQ-somatic well-being scores between the baseline (Week 0) and the endpoint (Week 6) were observed in the patients by ITT analysis.

Fourth, low baseline folate (≤5.65) or vitamin B12 (≤148.1) levels or elevated homocysteine levels (≥13.2) among the patients were not associated with the positive clinical response to the SAMe augmentation in this study. Aditionally, differences of mean levels of folate, vitamin B12, or homocysteine could not be observed between the responding patients and nonresponding patients to SAMe augmentation.

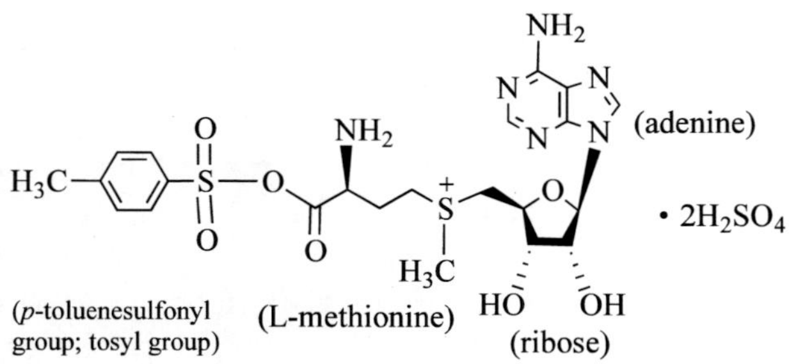

S-Adenosyl-L-methionine sulfate tosylate (SAMe-sulfate tosylate. **38**)

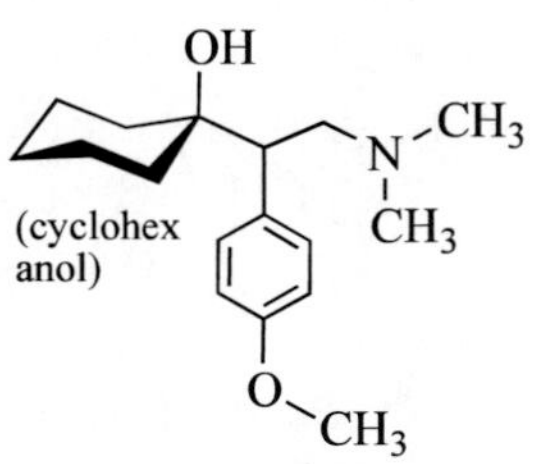

venlafaxine (**39**)

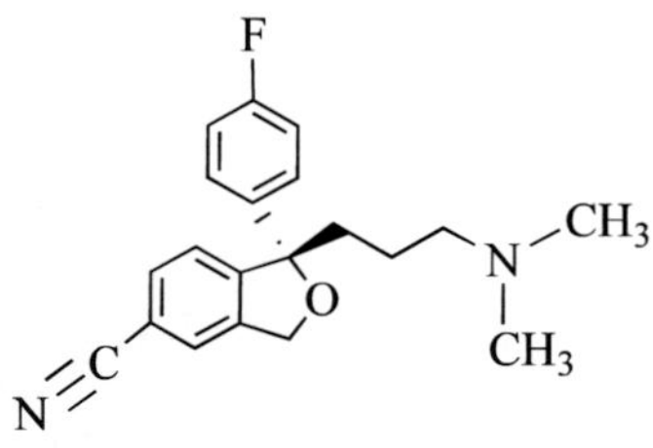

escitalopram (**40**)

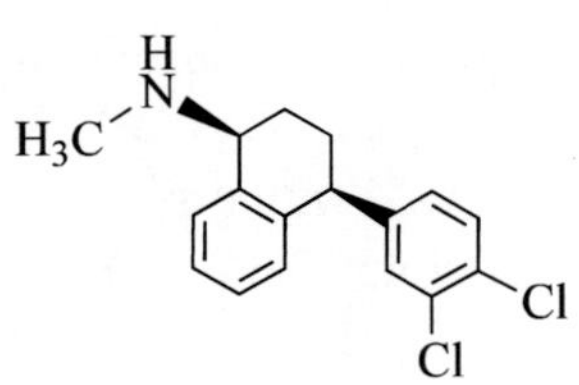

sertraline (**41**)

Figure 17. *S*-Adenosyl-L-methionine tosylate (SAMe-tosylate. **38**), venlafaxine (**39**), escitalopram (**40**) and sertraline (**41**).

Fifth, on the common adverse effect of *S*-adenosyl-L-methionine tosylate (SAMe-tosylate) 800-1,600 mg/d using 30 patients, gastrointestinal side effects were 50.0% for constipation, 16.6% for gastrointestinal upset, 16.6% for diarrhea/gas, and 6.6% for decreased appetite. Musculoskeletal/nervous side effects were 13.3% for headaches, 10.0% for activation (anxiety, irritability), 10.0% for fatigue and sedation, and 6.6% for sleep disturbance.

Results (First-Fifth) show the combination enhancement effect of SSRIs or venlafaxine with SAMe in a placebo-controlled trial in resistant depression. This means that the combined administration of SAMe with antidepressants provides a treatment technique for treatment-resistant depression (TRD) [38].

CONCLUSION

Nutraceuticals is a term newly coined word from nutrition plus pharmaceuticals; there are also many proposed definitions of nutraceuticals. I propose that nutraceuticals be divided into four parts. First is functional foods like USDA-approved foods, colored foods, and probiotic foods, Second is dietary supplements (nutritional supplements) like vitamin and mineral supplements, herbal supplements such as Ayurvedic herbal extracts, plant extracts, and plant protein supplements like protein powder, and healthy living lifestyle products. Third is functional beverages such as sports drinks and fortified juices, energy drinks, RTD teas, enhanced fruit drinks, soy beverages, and enhanced water. Fourth is natural phamaceuticals such as natural-substance derived antibacterial agents and discoloration and oxidation inhibitors for foods derived from natural products.

Psychiatric disorders include mental illnesses such as schizophrenia, mood disorders like depression and bipolar disorder, neurosis, dementia, epilepsy, sleeping disorder, and juvenile psychiatric disorders. Psychotropic drugs (psychoactive drug or minor tranquilizer) and antipsychotic drugs (major tranquilizer) can produce side effects including hypotension, arrhythmia, anorexia, nausea, diarrhea, constipation, headache, insomnia, fatigue, liver function failure, stomatitis, heart failure, frequent urination, dizziness, anxiety, decrease of attention and concentration. Plant-derived components generally show fewer adverse effects compared to the adverse effects of synthetic drugs. Many medicinal plants have been used in the prevention and treatment of depression and chizophrenia.

Omega-3 fatty acids (ω-3 FAs) such as DPA, DHA, LA, and AA have shown an improvement effect for schizophrenia. Sugar alcohol inositol, a sixfold alcohol (polyol) of cyclohexane, showed an improvement effect for panic disorder and depression, and combined administration of inositol with SSRI or serotonin enhanced the antidepressant effect. Folate and leucovorin are involved in folate deficiency during early neurodevelopment predisposed to schizophrenia. SAMe in naturally occurring food plant components showed from clinical meta-analysis a significant effect in treatment of depression.

This chapter reviewed the enhancement effect by combined administration of conventional psychotropic medicines or antipsychotic drugs with plant-derived components such as omega-3 fatty acids, inositol, folate, leucovorin, and SAMe for improvement and treament of depression and schizophrenia.

REFERENCES

[1] Brower V. Nutraceuticals: poised for a healthy slice of the healthcare market? *Nat Biotechnol* 16(8), 728-731, 1998.

[2] Kalra EK. Nutraceutical: definition and introduction. *AAPS PharmSci* 5(3), E25, 2003.

[3] Sunitha D, Chary MNK, Hemalatha K, Unissa R. a review on nutraceuticals. *Int J Pharm Res Bio-Sci* 5(1), 123-135, 2016.

[4] Palthur MP, Palthur SSS, Chitta SK. Nutraceuticals: a conceptual definition. *Int J Pharmacy Pharm Sc*i 2(3), 19-27, 2010.

[5] Sapkale AP, Thorat MS, Vir PR, Singh MC. Nutraceuticals: global status and applications: a review. *Int J Pharm Chem Sci* 1(3), 1166-1181, 2012.

[6] Borkar N, Saurabh SS, Rathore KS, Pandit A, Khandelwal KR. An insight on nutraceuticals. *PharmaTutor* 3(8), 13-23, 2015.

[7] Chauhan B, Kumar G, Kalam N, Ansari SH. Current concepts and prospects of herbal nutraceutical: a review. *J Adv Pharm Technol Res* 4(1), 4-8, 2013.

[8] Nasri H, Baradaran A, Shirzad H, Rafieian-Kopaei M. New concepts in nutraceuticals as alternative for pharmaceuticals. *Int J Prev Med* 5(12), 1487-1499, 2014.

[9] Ratnaparkhi PK, Karode NP, Patil KB, Gohel SN, Prajapati VD, Jani GK. Nutraceuticals: its current scenario and challenges in dietary supplements. *World J Pharm Pharmaceut Sci* 4(7), 460-474, 2015.

[10] Bhowmik D, Gopinath H, Kumar BP, Duraivel S, Kumar KPS. Nutraceutical: a bright scope and opportunity of Indian healthcare market. *The Pharma Innovation J* 1(11), 29-41, 2013.

[11] Sunitha D, Chary MNK, Hemalatha K, Unissa R. A review on nutraceuticals. *Int J Pharm Res Bio-Sci* 5(1), 123-135, 2016.

[12] Murray CJ, Lopez AD. Alternative projections of mortality and disability by cause 1990-2020: global burden of disease study. *Lancet* 349(9064), 1498-1504, 1997.

[13] Bozzatello P, Brignolo E, De Grandi E, Bellino S. Supplementation with omega-3 fatty acids in psychiatric disorders: a review of literature data. *J Clin Med* 5(8), pii.E67, 2016.

[14] United States Department of Agriculture Agricultural Research Service. *National Nutrient Database for Standard Reference Release 28.* Released 2015, rev. 2016. https://ndb.nal.usda.gov/ndb/search/list.

[15] Yehuda S, Rabinovitz S, Mostofsky DI. Essential fatty acids are mediators of brain biochemistry and cognitive functions. *J Neurosci Res* 56(6), 565-570, 1999.

[16] Salem N. Omega-3 fatty acids: molecular and biochemical aspects. In: Spilier G, Scala J (eds). *New Protective Role for Selected Nutrients.* 1989. Alan R. Liss, Inc., New York. 109-228.

[17] Assisi A1, Banzi R, Buonocore C, Capasso F, Di Muzio V, Michelacci F, Renzo D, Tafuri G, Trotta F, Vitocolonna M, Garattini S. Fish oil and mental health: the role of n-3 long-chain polyunsaturated fatty acids in cognitive development and neurological disorders. *Int Clin Psychopharmacol* 21(6), 319-336, 2006.

[18] Roy A, Virkkunen M, Linnoila M. Serotonin in suicide, violence, and alcoholism. In: Coccaro E, Murphy P (eds). *Serotonin in Major Psychiatric Disorders.* 1991. American Psychiatric Press, Washington, DC. 187-208.

[19] Hibbeln JR, Linnoila M, Umhau JC, Rawlings R, George DT, Salem N Jr. Essential fatty acids predict metabolites of serotonin and dopamine in cerebrospinal fluid among healthy control subjects, and early- and late-onset alcoholics. *Biol Psychiatry* 44(4), 235-242, 1998.

[20] Stanley M, Traskman-Bendz L, Dorovini-Zis K. Correlations between aminergic metabolites simultaneously obtained from human CSF and brain. *Life Sci* 37(14), 1279-1286, 1985.

[21] Mann JJ. Violence and aggression: 1919-1928. In: Bloom FE, Kupfer DJ (eds). *Psychopharmacology: The Fourth Generation of Progress.* 1995. Raven Press, New York.

[22] Virkkunen M, Rawlings R, Tokola R, Poland RE, Guidotti A, Nemeroff C, Bissette G, Kalogeras K, Karonen SL, Linnoila M. CSF biochemistries, glucose metabolism, and diurnal activity rhythms in alcoholic, violent offenders, fire setters, and healthy volunteers. *Arch Gen Psychiatry* 51(1), 20-27, 1994.

[23] Linnoila M, Virkkunen M, Scheinin M, Nuutila A, Rimon R, Goodwin FK. Low cerebrospinal fluid 5-hydroxyindoleacetic acid concentration differentiates impulsive from nonimpulsive violent behavior. *Life Sci* 33(26), 2609-2614, 1983.

[24] Muldoon MF, Manuck SB, Matthews KA. Lowering cholesterol concentrations and mortality: a quantitative review of primary prevention trials. *BMJ* 301(6747), 309-314, 1990.

[25] Engelberg H. Low serum cholesterol and suicide. *Lancet* 339(8795), 727-729, 1992.

[26] Kaplan JR, Shively CA, Fontenot MB, Morgan TM, Howell SM, Manuck SB, Muldoon MF, Mann JJ. Demonstration of an association among dietary cholesterol, central serotonergic activity, and social behavior in monkeys. *Psychosom Med* 56(6), 479-484, 1994.

[27] Salem N Jr, Kim HY, Yergey JA. Docosahexaenoic acid: Membrane function and metabolism. In: Simopoulos A, Kifer RR, Martin R (eds). *Health Effects of Polyunsaturated Fatty Acids in Seafoods*. 1986. Academic Press, New York. 263-317.

[28] Yergey JA, Kim HY, Salem N Jr. High-performance liquid chromatography/thermospray mass spectrometry of eicosanoids and novel oxygenated metabolites of docosahexaenoic acid. *Anal Chem* 58(7), 1344-1348, 1986.

[29] Virkkunen ME, Horrobin DF, Jenkins DK, Manku MS. Plasma phospholipid essential fatty acids and prostaglandins in alcoholic, habitually violent, and impulsive offenders. *Biol Psychiatry* 22(9), 1087-1096, 1987.

[30] Farquharson J, Cockburn F, Patrick WA, Jamieson EC, Logan RW. Infant cerebral cortex phospholipid fatty-acid composition and diet. *Lancet* 340(8823), 810-813, 1992.

[31] Hibbeln JR, Umhau JC, Linnoila M, George DT, Ragan PW, Shoaf SE, Vaughan MR, Rawlings R, Salem N Jr. A replication study of violent and nonviolent subjects: cerebrospinal fluid metabolites of serotonin and dopamine are predicted by plasma essential fatty acids. *Biol Psychiatry* 44(4), 243-249, 1998.

[32] Edwards R, Peet M, Shay J, Horrobin D. Omega-3 polyunsaturated fatty acid levels in the diet and in red blood cell membranes of depressed patients. *J Affect Disord* 48(2-3), 149-155, 1998.

[33] Nemets B, Stahl ZM, Belmaker RH. Addition of omega-3 fatty acid to maintenance medication treatment for recurrent unipolar depressive disorder. *Am J Psychiatry* 159(3), 477-479, 2002.

[34] Hibbeln JR, Salem N Jr. Dietary polyunsaturated fatty acids and depression: when cholesterol does not satisfy. *Am J Clin Nutr* 62(1), 1-9, 1995.

[35] Stoll AL, Severus WE, Freeman MP, Rueter S, Zboyan HA, Diamond E, Cress KK, Marangell LB. Omega 3 fatty acids in bipolar disorder: a preliminary double-blind, placebo-controlled trial. *Arch Gen Psychiatry* 56(5), 407-412, 1999.

[36] Maes M, Christophe A, Delanghe J, Altamura C, Neels H, Meltzer HY. Lowered omega 3 polyunsaturated fatty acids in serum phospholipids and cholesteryl esters of depressed patients. *Psychiatry Res* 85(3), 275-291, 1999.

[37] Severus WE, Ahrens B, Stoll AL. Omega-3 fatty acids: the missing link? *Arch Gen Psychiatry* 56(4), 380-381, 1999.

[38] Alpert JE, Papakostas G, Mischoulon D, Worthington JJ 3rd, Petersen T, Mahal Y, Burns A, Bottiglieri T, Nierenberg AA, Fava M. *S*-adenosyl-L-methionine (SAMe) as an adjunct for resistant major depressive disorder: an open trial following partial or nonresponse to selective serotonin reuptake inhibitors or venlafaxine. *J Clin Psychopharmacol* 24(6), 661-664, 2004.

[39] Franzini A, Messina G, Marras C, Savino M, Miniati M, Bugiani O, Broggi G. Hamilton rating scale for depression: 21 modifications in patients with vagal nerve stimulation for treatment of treatment-resistant depression: series report. *Neuromodulation* 11(4), 267-271, 2008.

[40] Hashimoto M. Improvement effect of docosahexaenoic acid on neurological function and its application to neurological disorders. *Oleoscience* 6(2), 67-76, 2006. In Japanese.

[41] Su KP, Huang SY, Chiu CC, Shen WW. Omega-3 fatty acids in major depressive disorder: a preliminary double-blind, placebo-controlled trial. *Eur Neuropsychopharmacol* 13(4), 267-271, 2003.

[42] Hoen WP, Lijmer JG, Duran M, Wanders RJ, van Beveren NJ, de Haan L. Red blood cell polyunsaturated fatty acids measured in red blood cells and schizophrenia: a meta-analysis. *Psychiatry Res* 207(1-2), 1-12, 2013.

[43] Pawełczyk T, Grancow M, Kotlicka-Antczak M, Trafalska E, Gębski P, Szemraj J, Żurner N, Pawełczyk A. Omega-3 fatty acids in first-episode schizophrenia: a randomized controlled study of efficacy and relapse prevention (OFFER): rationale, design, and methods. *BMC Psychiatry* 15(97), 2015.

[44] Agostoni C. Role of long-chain polyunsaturated fatty acids in the first year of life. *J Pediatr Gastroenterol Nutr* 47(Suppl 2), S41-S44, 2008.

[45] Singh M. Essential fatty acids, DHA and human brain. *Indian J Pediatr* 72(3), 239-242, 2005.

[46] Beydoun MA, Kaufman JS, Sloane PD, Heiss G, Ibrahim J. n-3 fatty acids, hypertension and risk of cognitive decline among older adults in the Atherosclerosis Risk in Communities (ARIC) study. *Public Health Nutr* 11(1), 17-29, 2008.

[47] Katon W, Rutter C, Ludman EJ, Von Korff M, Lin E, Simon G, Bush T, Walker E, Unützer J. A randomized trial of relapse prevention of depression in primary care. *Arch Gen Psychiatry* 58(3), 241-247, 2001.

[48] Liberman RP, Kopelowicz A. Sustained remission of schizophrenia. *Am J Psychiatry* 162(9), 1763-1764, 2005. Author reply.

[49] Jääskeläinen E, Juolal P, Hirvonen N, McGrath JJ, Saha S, Isohanni M, Veijolal J, Miettunen J. Systematic review and meta-analysis of recovery in schizophrenia. *Schizophr Bull* 2012.

[50] Lieberman JA, Stroup TS, Perkins DO (eds). *The American Psychiatric Publishing Textbook of Schizophrenia.* 2006. American Psychiatric Publishing, Washington, DC.

[51] Alvarez-Jimenez M, Priede A, Hetrick SE, Bendall S, Killackey E, Parker AG, McGorry PD, Gleeson JF. Risk factors for relapse following treatment for first episode psychosis: a systematic review and meta-analysis of longitudinal studies. *Schizophr Res* 139(1-3), 116-128, 2012.

[52] Linszen D, Dingemans P, Lenior M. Early intervention and a five year follow up in young adults with a short duration of untreated psychosis: ethical implications. *Schizophr Res* 51(1), 55-61, 2001.

[53] Emsley R, Chiliza B, Asmal L, Harvey BH. The nature of relapse in schizophrenia. *BMC Psychiatry* 13(50), 2013.

[54] Emsley R, Myburgh C, Oosthuizen P, van Rensburg SJ. Randomized, placebo-controlled study of ethyl-eicosapentaenoic acid as supplemental treatment in schizophrenia. *Am J Psychiatry* 159(9), 1596-1598, 2002.

[55] Emsley R, Niehaus DJ, Koen L, Oosthuizen PP, Turner HJ, Carey P, van Rensburg SJ, Maritz JS, Murck H. The effects of eicosapentaenoic acid in tardive dyskinesia: a randomized, placebo-controlled trial. *Schizophr Res* 84(1), 112-120, 2006.

[56] Berger GE, Proffitt TM, McConchie M, Yuen H, Wood SJ, Amminger GP, Brewer W, McGorry PD. Ethyl-eicosapentaenoic acid in first-episode psychosis: a randomized, placebo-controlled trial. *J Clin Psychiatry* 68(12), 1867-1875, 2007.

[57] Pisano S, Gritti A, Catone G, Pascotto A. Antipsychotic-induced dyslipidemia treated with omega 3 fatty acid supplement in an 11-year-old psychotic child: a 1-year follow-up. *J Child Adolesc Psychopharmacol* 23(2), 139-141, 2013.

[58] Faghihi T, Jahed A, Mahmoudi-Gharaei J, Sharifi V, Akhondzadeh S, Ghaeli P. Role of Omega-3 fatty acids in preventing metabolic disturbances in patients on olanzapine plus either sodium valproate or lithium: a randomized double-blind placebo-controlled trial. *Daru* 20(1), 43, 2012.

[59] Barcelos RC, Benvegnú DM, Boufleur N, Reckziegel P, Müller LG, Pase C, Emanuelli T, Bürger ME. Effects of omega-3 essential fatty acids (omega-3 EFAs) on motor disorders and memory dysfunction typical neuroleptic-induced: behavioral and biochemical parameter. *Neurotox Res* 17(3), 228-237, 2010.

[60] Sarsilmaz M, Songur A, Ozyurt H, Kuş I, Ozen OA, Ozyurt B, Söğüt S, Akyol O. Potential role of dietary omega-3 essential fatty acids on some oxidant/antioxidant parameters in rats' corpus striatum. *Prostaglandins Leukot Essent Fatty Acids* 69(4), 253-259, 2003.

[61] Cardoso HD, dos Santos Junior EF, de Santana DF, Gonçalves-Pimentel C, Angelim MK, Isaac AR, Lagranha CJ, Guedes RC, Beltrão EI, Morya E, Rodrigues MC, Andrade-da-Costa BL. Omega-3 deficiency and neurodegeneration in the substantia nigra: involvement of increased nitric oxide production and reduced BDNF expression. *Biochim Biophys Acta* 1840(6), 1902-1912, 2014.

[62] Alvarez-Jiménez M, Parker AG, Hetrick SE, McGorry PD, Gleeson JF. Preventing the second episode: a systematic review and meta-analysis of psychosocial and pharmacological trials in first-episode psychosis. *Schizophr Bull* 37(3), 619-630, 2011.

[63] Andreasen NC, Liu D, Ziebell S, Vora A, Ho BC. Relapse duration, treatment intensity, and brain tissue loss in schizophrenia: a prospective longitudinal MRI study. *Am J Psychiatry* 170(6), 609-615, 2013.

[64] Emsley R, Chiliza B, Asmal L, du Plessis S, Phahladira L, van Niekerk E, van Rensburg SJ, Harvey BH. A randomized, controlled trial of omega-3 fatty acids plus an antioxidant for relapse prevention after antipsychotic discontinuation in first-episode schizophrenia. *Schizophr Res* 158(1-3), 230-235, 2014.

[65] Harper KN, Hibbeln JR, Deckelbaum R, Quesenberry CP Jr, Schaefer CA, Brown AS. Maternal serum docosahexaenoic acid and schizophrenia spectrum disorders in adult offspring. *Schizophr Res* 128(1-3), 30-36, 2011.

[66] Rogers LK, Valentine CJ, Keim SA. DHA supplementation: current implications in pregnancy and childhood. *Pharmacol Res* 70(1), 13-19, 2013.

[67] Zugno AI, Chipindo HL, Volpato AM, Budni J, Steckert AV, de Oliveira MB, Heylmann AS, da Rosa Silveira F, Mastella GA, Maravai SG, Wessler PG, Binatti AR, Panizzutti B, Schuck PF, Quevedo J, Gama CS. Omega-3 prevents behavior response and brain oxidative damage in the ketamine model of schizophrenia. *Neuroscience* 259, 223-231, 2014.

[68] Cederholm T, Salem N Jr, Palmblad J. ω-3 fatty acids in the prevention of cognitive decline in humans. *Adv Nutr* 4(6), 672-676, 2013.

[69] Janssen CI, Kiliaan AJ. Long-chain polyunsaturated fatty acids (LCPUFA) from genesis to senescence: the influence of LCPUFA on neural development, aging, and neurodegeneration. *Prog Lipid Res* 53, 1-17, 2014.

[70] Budavari S (ed). *The Merck Index*, 11th ed. 1989. Merck & Co., Inc..

[71] Holland B, Unwin ID, Buss DH (eds). *Fruit and Nuts: First Supplement to the Fifth Edition of McCance and Widdowson's The Composition of Foods*. 1992. Royal Society of Chemistry, Ministry of Agriculture, Fisheries and Food. The Bath Press, UK.

[72] Clements RS Jr, Darnell B. Myo-inositol content of common foods: development of a high-myo-inositol diet. *Am J Clin Nutr* 33(9), 1954-1967, 1980.

[73] Parfitt K, Martindale W. *Martindale: The Complete Drug Reference, 32nd ed.* 1999. Pharmaceutical Press, London, UK.

[74] Barkai AI, Dunner DL, Gross HA, Mayo P, Fieve RR. Reduced myo-inositol levels in cerebrospinal fluid from patients with affective disorder. *Biol Psychiatry* 13(1), 65-72, 1978.

[75] Levine J, Gonsalves M, Babur I, Belmaker RH. Inositol 6 gm daily may be effective in depression but not schizophrenia. *Human Psychopharmacology Clinical and Experimenta*l 8(1), 49-53, 1993.

[76] Levine J, Barak Y, Gonzalves M, Szor H, Elizur A, Kofman O, Belmaker R. Double-blind, controlled trial of inositol treatment of depression. *Am J Psychiatry* 152(5), 792-794, 1995.

[77] Belmaker RH, Jevine J. Inositol in treatment of psychiatric disorders. In: Mischoulon D, Rosenbaum JF (eds). *Natural Medications for Psychiatric Disorders: Considering the Alternatives, 2nd ed.* 2008. Lippincott, Williams and Wilkins, Baltimore, MD. 105-115.

[78] Benjamin J, Levine J, Fux M, Aviv A, Levy D, Belmaker RH. Double-blind, placebo-controlled, crossover trial of inositol treatment for panic disorder. *Am J Psychiatry* 152(7), 1084-1086, 1995.

[79] Levine J. Controlled trials of inositol in psychiatry. *Eur Neuropsychopharmacol* 7(2), 147-155, 1997.

[80] Levine J, Mishori A, Susnosky M, Martin M, Belmaker RH. Combination of inositol and serotonin reuptake inhibitors in the treatment of depression. *Biol Psychiatry* 45(3), 270-273, 1999.

[81] Tumati S, Martens S, Aleman A. Magnetic resonance spectroscopy in mild cognitive impairment: systematic review and meta-analysis. *Neurosci Biobehav Rev* 37(10 part 2), 2571-2586, 2013.

[82] Kantarci K. Proton MRS in mild cognitive impairment. *J Magn Reson Imaging* 37(4), 770-777, 2013.

[83] Coupland NJ, Ogilvie CJ, Hegadoren KM, Seres P, Hanstock CC, Allen PS. Decreased prefrontal myo-inositol in major depressive disorder. *Biol Psychiatry* 57(12), 1526-1534, 2005.

[84] Fenili D, Brown M, Rappaport R, McLaurin J. Properties of scyllo-inositol as a therapeutic treatment of AD-like pathology. *J Mol Med (Berl)* 85(6), 603-611, 2007.

[85] Dickson DW. The pathogenesis of senile plaques. *J Neuropathol Exp Neurol* 56(4), 321-339, 1997.

[86] Wang HW, Pasternak JF, Kuo H, Ristic H, Lambert MP, Chromy B, Viola KL, Klein WL, Stine WB, Krafft GA, Trommer BL. Soluble oligomers of beta amyloid (1-42) inhibit long-term potentiation but not long-term depression in rat dentate gyrus. *Brain Res* 924(2), 133-140, 2002.

[87] Shonk TK, Moats RA, Gifford P, Michaelis T, Mandigo JC, Izumi J, Ross BD. Probable Alzheimer disease: diagnosis with proton MR spectroscopy. *Radiology* 195(1), 65-72, 1995.

[88] Choi JK, Carreras I, Dedeoglu A, Jenkins BG. Detection of increased scyllo-inositol in brain with magnetic resonance spectroscopy after dietary supplementation in Alzheimer's disease mouse models. *Neuropharmacology* 59(4-5), 353-357, 2010.

[89] Susser ES, Lin SP. Schizophrenia after prenatal exposure to the Dutch Hunger Winter of 1944-1945. *Arch Gen Psychiatry* 49(12), 983-988, 1992.

[90] Jones P. Schizophrenia after prenatal exposure to the Dutch hunger winter of 1944-1945. *Arch Gen Psychiatry* 51(4), 333-334, 1994.

[91] Brown AS, Susser ES, Butler PD, Richardson Andrews R, Kaufmann CA, Gorman JM. Neurobiological plausibility of prenatal nutritional deprivation as a risk factor for schizophrenia. *J Nerv Ment Dis* 184(2), 71-85, 1996.

[92] Morgane PJ, Austin-LaFrance R, Bronzino J, Tonkiss J, Díaz-Cintra S, Cintra L, Kemper T, Galler JR. Prenatal malnutrition and development of the brain. *Neurosci Biobehav Rev* 17(1), 91-128, 1993.

[93] Butler PD, Susser ES, Brown AS, Charles A Kaufman CA, Gorman JM. Prenatal nutritional deprivation as a risk factor in schizophrenia: preclinical evidence. *Neuropsychopharmacol* 11(4), 227-235, 1994.

[94] Stein Z, Susser M, Saenger G, Marolla F (eds). *Famine and Human Development: Dutch Hunger Winter of 1944-45*. 1975. Oxford Medicine Publications, UK.

[95] Done DJ, Johnstone EC, Frith CD, Golding J, Shepherd PM, Crow TJ. Complications of pregnancy and delivery in relation to psychosis in adult life: data from the British perinatal mortality survey sample. *BMJ* 302(6792), 1576-1580, 1991.

[96] Wiersma D, Giel R, De Jong A, Slooff CJ. Social class and schizophrenia in a Dutch cohort. *Psychol Med* 13(1), 141-150, 1983.

[97] MRC Vitamin Study Research Group. Prevention of neural tube defects: results of the Medical Research Council Vitamin Study. *Lancet* 338(8760), 131-137, 1991.

[98] Czeizel AE, Dudás I. Prevention of the first occurrence of neural-tube defects by periconceptional vitamin supplementation. *N Engl J Med* 327(26), 1832-1835, 1992.

[99] Elwood JM, Little J. *Epidemiology and control of neural tube defects.* 1993. Monographs in Epidemiology and Biostatistics. Oxford University Press, New York.

[100] Susser E, Neugebauer R, Hoek HW, Brown AS, Lin S, Labovitz D, Gorman JM. Schizophrenia after prenatal famine: further evidence. *Arch Gen Psychiatry* 53(1), 25-31, 1996.

[101] Alpert JE, Mischoulon D, Rubenstein GE, Bottonari K, Nierenberg AA, Fava M. Folinic acid (leucovorin) as an adjunctive treatment for SSRI-refractory depression. *Ann Clin Psychiatry* 14(1), 33-38, 2002.

[102] Coppen A, Bailey J. Enhancement of the antidepressant action of fluoxetine by folic acid: a randomised, placebo controlled trial. *J Affect Disord* 60(2), 121-130, 2000.

[103] St Clair D, Xu M, Wang P, Yu Y, Fang Y, Zhang F, Zheng X, Gu N, Feng G, Sham P, He L. Rates of adult schizophrenia following prenatal exposure to the Chinese famine of 1959-1961. *JAMA* 294(5), 557-562, 2005.

[104] Miyamoto S, Duncan GE, Marx CE, Lieberman JA. Treatments for schizophrenia: a critical review of pharmacology and mechanisms of action of antipsychotic drugs. *Mol Psychiatry* 10(1), 79-104, 2005.

[105] Davey JW, Hohenlohe PA, Etter PD, Boone JQ, Catchen JM, Blaxter ML. Genome-wide genetic marker discovery and genotyping using next-generation sequencing. *Nat Rev Genet* 12(7), 499-510, 2011.

[106] Lencz T, Szeszko PR, DeRosse P, Burdick KE, Bromet EJ, Bilder RM, Malhotra AK. A schizophrenia risk gene, ZNF804A, influences neuroanatomical and neurocognitive phenotypes. *Neuropsychopharmacology* 35(11), 2284-2291, 2010.

[107] Amiel J, Rio M, de Pontual L, Redon R, Malan V, Boddaert N, Plouin P, Carter NP, Lyonnet S, Munnich A, Colleaux L. Mutations in TCF4, encoding a class I basic helix-loop-helix transcription factor, are responsible for Pitt-Hopkins syndrome, a severe epileptic encephalopathy associated with autonomic dysfunction. *Am J Hum Genet* 80(5), 988-993, 2007.

[108] Zweier C, Peippo MM, Hoyer J, Sousa S, Bottani A, Clayton-Smith J, Reardon W, Saraiva J, Cabral A, Gohring I, Devriendt K, de Ravel T, Bijlsma EK, Hennekam RC, Orrico A, Cohen M, Dreweke A, Reis A, Nurnberg P, Rauch A. Haploinsufficiency of TCF4 causes syndromal mental retardation with intermittent hyperventilation (Pitt-Hopkins syndrome). *Am J Hum Genet* 80(5), 994-1001, 2007.

[109] Sekar A, Bialas AR, de Rivera H, Davis A, Hammond TR, Kamitaki N, Tooley K, Presumey J, Baum M, Van Doren V, Genovese G, Rose SA, Handsaker RE, Daly MJ, Carroll MC, Stevens B, McCarroll SA; Schizophrenia Working Group of the Psychiatric Genomics Consortium. Schizophrenia risk from complex variation of complement component 4. *Nature* 530(7589), 177-183, 2016.

[110] Zhong L, Brown J, Kramer A, Kaleka K, Petersen A, Krueger JN, Florence M, Muelbl MJ, Battle M, Murphy GG, Olsen CM, Gerges NZ. Increased prefrontal cortex neurogranin enhances plasticity and extinction learning. *J Neurosci* 35(19), 7503-7508, 2015.

[111] Marshall CR, Scherer SW. Detection and characterization of copy number variation in autism spectrum disorder. *Methods Mol Biol* 838, 115-135, 2012.

[112] Van Winkel R, Esquivel G, Kenis G, Wichers M, Collip D, Peerbooms O, Rutten B, Myin-Germeys I, Van Os J. Review: genome-wide findings in schizophrenia and the role of gene-environment interplay. *CNS Neurosci Ther* 16(5), e185-e192, 2010.

[113] Hill M, Shannahan K, Jasinski S, Macklin EA, Raeke L, Roffman JL, Goff DC. Folate supplementation in schizophrenia: a possible role for MTHFR genotype. *Schizophr Res* 127(1-3), 41-45, 2011.

[114] Roffman JL, Lamberti JS, Achtyes E, Macklin EA, Galendez GC, Raeke LH, Silverstein NJ, Smoller JW, Hill M, Goff DC. Randomized multicenter investigation of folate plus vitamin B12 supplementation in schizophrenia. *JAMA Psychiatry* 70(5), 481-489, 2013.

[115] Linde K, Ramirez G, Mulrow CD, Pauls A, Weidenhammer W, Melchart D. St John's wort for depression: an overview and meta-analysis of randomised clinical trials. *BMJ* 313(7052), 253-258, 1996.

[116] Stevinson C, Ernst E. Hypericum for depression: an update of the clinical evidence. *Eur Neuropsychopharmacol* 9(6), 501-505, 1999.

[117] Kessler RC, Soukup J, Davis RB, Foster DF, Wilkey SA, Van Rompay MI, Eisenberg DM. The use of complementary and alternative therapies to treat anxiety and depression in the United States. *Am J Psychiatry* 158(2), 289-294, 2001.

[118] Cantoni GL. The nature of the active methyl donor formed enzymatically from L-methionine and adenosinetriphosphate. *J Am Chem Soc* 74 (11), 2942–2943, 1952.

[119] Bottiglieri T. *S*-Adenosyl-L-methionine (SAMe): from the bench to the bedside: molecular basis of a pleiotrophic molecule. *Am J Clin Nutr* 76(5), 1151S-1157S, 2002.

[120] Resources Council, Science and Technology Agency. *Standard Tables of Food Composition in Japan: Amino Acid Composition of Foods*, rev. ed., 1986.

[121] Bressa GM. *S*-adenosyl-l-methionine (SAMe) as antidepressant: meta-analysis of clinical studies. *Acta Neurol Scand Suppl* 154, 7-14, 1994.

In: Nutraceuticals
Editor: Noboru Motohashi
ISBN: 978-1-53611-785-1

Chapter 2

COMMON BEANS (*PHASEOLUS VULGARIS*): A BRIEF DESCRIPTION OF NUTRITIONAL AND NUTRACEUTICAL PROFILES FOR POTENTIAL WEIGHT-CONTROL APPLICATIONS

Lourdes Valadez-Carmona[1], *Carla Patricia Plazola-Jacinto*[1], *Marcela Hernández-Ortega*[2] *and Gabriela Gutiérrez-Salmeán*[2,*]

[1]Departamento de Ingeniería Bioquímica, Escuela Nacional de Ciencias Biológicas, Instituto Politécnico Nacional, México
[2]Facultad de Ciencias de la Salud, Universidad Anáhuac México (Campus Norte), México

* Corresponding author Email: gabrielasalmean@yahoo.com; Telephone: (52) (55) 5627 0210 Ext. 7230; Address: Dr. Gabriela Gutiérrez-Salmeán, Facultad de Ciencias de la Salud. Universidad Anáhuac México, Campus Norte, Av. Universidad Anáhuac #46. Lomas Anáhuac. Huixquilucan, Estado de México. 52786. México.

ABSTRACT

Beans have been consumed since prehispanic times and, nowadays, are one of the most eaten legumes worldwide. Among ~70 varieties, beans are now considered as functional foods due to the presence of different phytochemicals, e.g., phenolic compounds. These have been reported to exhibit a wide variety of nutraceutic effects, including those oriented to weight-control and therefore, obesity.

Although evidence of both observational and experimental studies has revealed positive tendencies related to bean consumption/ supplementation and weight-loss, more rigorous trials are needed in order to consider this functional food within the every-day therapeutics of obesity.

Keywords: beans, functional foods, nutraceuticals, obesity, overweight, *Phaseolus vulgaris,* phytochemicals

ABBREVIATIONS

α-linolenic acid (1)
eicosapentanoic acid (EPA. 2)
docosahexaenoic acid (DHA. 3)
phytic acid (4)
kaempferol (5)
delphinidin (6)
gallic acid (7)
anillic acid (8)
caffeic acid (9)
coumaric acid (10)
ferulic acid acid (11)
kaempferol-3-*O*-glucoside (12)
pelargonidin 3-glucoside (13)
quercetin (14)
daidzein (15)
genistein (16)
isorhamnetin (17)
naringenin(18)
propionic (19)

butyric acid (20)
sucrose (21)
raffinose (22)
stachyose (23)
verbascose (24)
α-AI: α-amylase inhibitors
BMI: body mass index
CCK: cholecystokinin
E-PHA: erythroagglutinating phytohemagglutinin
FAS: fatty acid synthase
GLP-1: glucagon-like peptide-1
HAs: hemagglutinins
HIV-1: human immunodeficiency virus type 1
iNOS: inducible nitric oxide synthase
JAK2: Janus kinase 2
L-PHA: leukoagglutinating phytohemagglutinin
LPS: lipopolysaccharide
NF-κB: NF-kappa-B
NDC: National Drug Code
NO: nitric oxide
PHA: phytohemagglutinin
PVE: *P. vulgaris* dry extracts
RFO: raffinose family of oligosaccharides
SCFA: short chain fatty acids
STAT-1: signal transducer and activator of transcription 1

1. Introduction

The common bean (*Phaseolus vulgaris* L.) was originally domesticated in Mesoamerica –mainly in the current territories of Mexico, Guatemala, Peru- as early as 6000 BC. In fact, it was part of a traditional prehispanic agrosystem –called *milpa*- which was composed of "the three sisters": beans, maize (corn), and squash (*Cucurbita pepo*) –sometimes chile (*Capsicum* L.) was also incorporated-. Nowadays, it is one of the most important food legumes, consumed worldwide as either a vegetable or a pulse (i.e., pods of green beans or as seeds of dry beans, respectively).

This widely accepted food provides significant advantages, not only because of its high-quality nutritional contents (e.g., rich and –generally- inexpensive source of protein, complex carbohydrates, minerals, vitamins, and dietary fiber) but for the nutraceutical (due to its contents of a wide variety of phytochemicals) potential and the health benefits (e.g., reduced risk of gastrointestinal and cardiovascular disease, diabetes mellitus, obesity, and some types of cancer), it has been consistently been associated to. As it happens, common beans have been an important part of folklore culture and applied within traditional medicine for treating diverse conditions: from rheumatism, acne and burns to diarrhea, dysentery and eczema [1].

As non-communicable chronic diseases -including obesity- have risen, common beans –which have shown, in observational studies, a positive association between their dietary consumption and a reduced risk for some of these diseases-[2] have gained increasing attention as a *functional food* [3, 4] with potential applications within the therapeutics of weight control.

2. Nutritional Profile

The common bean is a member of the *Phaseoulus* genus within the *Fabaceae* family, has been traditionally cultivated for its edible seeds –either dried or green-; however, its leaves and straw are sometimes also consumed [2].

Beans are considered a highly nutritious food: a serving of 100 g yields ~350 kcal thus are calorie-dense [5]. But, moreover, beans are often called "meat of the poor," mainly due to its protein content and quality: a little over 20% of its dry weight, with methionine being the limiting amino acid (therefore legumes are often recommended to be consumed with cereals, as they complement each other's protein profile) [2].

Although the main macronutrient in beans are carbohydrates (up to 65% of its total caloric content), these are considered to have a low-glycemic index and, moreover, contribute to the reduction of the correspondent indexes of other foods, i.e., lower the glycemic load of the complete meal. In addition, beans are a good source of dietary fiber (15 g/100 g), which not only prevents/helps treating constipation but also acts as a prebiotic –due to its content of resistant starches: stachyose and raffinose [6].

Regarding micronutrient profile, beans are good dietary sources of calcium and iron, but also zinc, potassium, phosphorous, and magnesium; vitamin B complex (particularly folates) [2, 7].

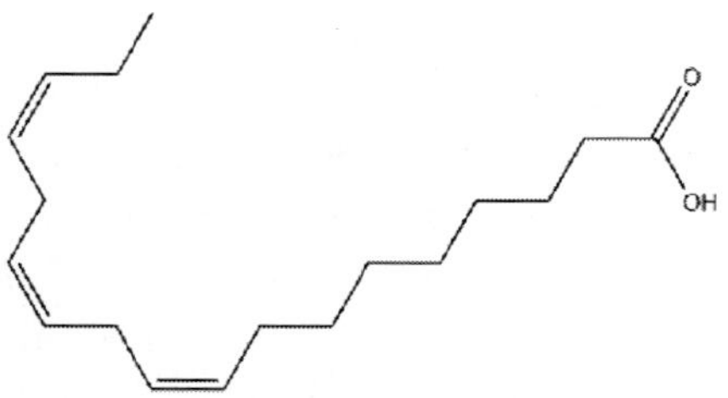

α-linolenic acid (1)

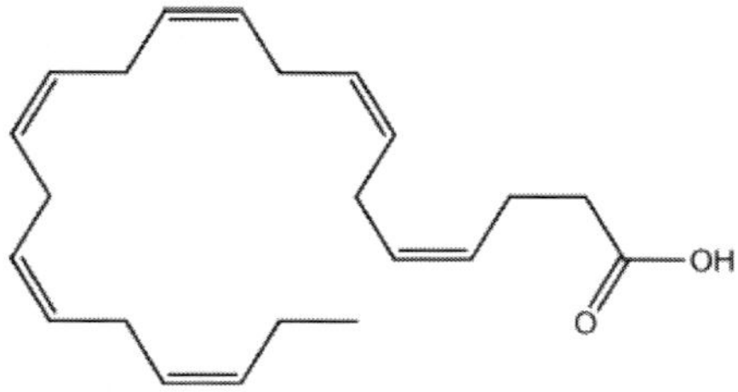

eicosapentanoic acid (EPA. 2)

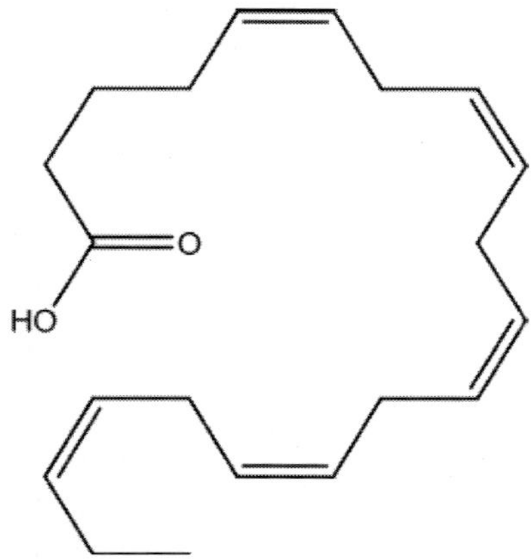

docosahexaenoic acid (DHA. 3)

Figure 1. α-Linolenic acid (1), eicosapentanoic acid (EPA. 2), and docosahexaenoic acid (DHA. 3).

And although the lipid fraction of is fairly low (~1.5% of its dry weight), common beans contain α-linolenic acid (1) (Figure 1) –an omega-3 which is metabolized into eicosapentanoic and docosahexaenoic fatty acids ((2) and (3)) (Figure 1) that have been proved to exert anti-inflammatory effects thus have been associated with a decreased cardiovascular and metabolic overall risk [2].

2.1. Antinutrients

Although bean seeds are, due to the aforementioned, considered as highly nutritious foods, they have also been reported to contain certain substances known as *antinutrients*, which can exert negative effects, ranging from broad toxicity and causing undesirable physiological effects (e.g., flatulence) to the interaction and further inhibition (or decrease in) of absorption/metabolism/ excretion on other nutrients (e.g., minerals, proteins) [8–10].

Some of these antinutrients include: oligosaccharides such as α-galactosides of sucrose, phytic acid (4) (Figure 2), protease inhibitors, lectins and saponines as well some condensed tannins and polyphenols. Nevertheless, recent epidemiological and experimental studies have demonstrated that many of these considered antinutrients may actually have beneficial effects (particularly polyphenols, saponins, tannins, *etc.*) Thus, they can be considered as nutrients and/or pronutrients with deleterious and/or beneficial effects on health depending of their specific chemical structure, concentration, overall consumption in diet but, moreover, depending in the specific interaction being analyzed within a specific clinical scenario (e.g., as saponins form complexes with dietary cholesterol, they could be considered as deleterious if the study subject were undernourished; in contrast, they should be considered as exhibiting a beneficial effect whereas the subject presented hypercholesterolemia [8, 11, 12].

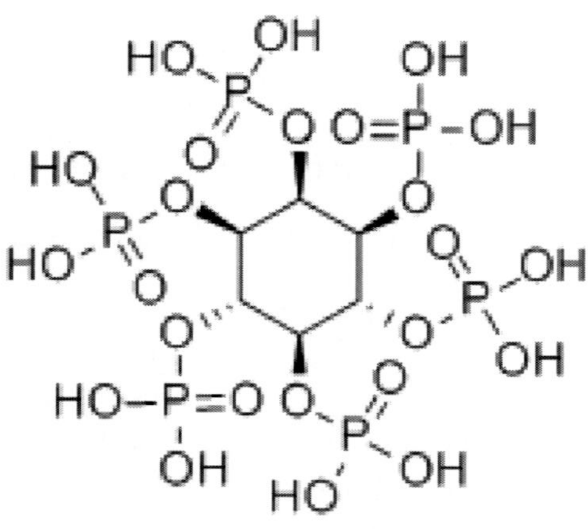

phytic acid (4)

Figure 2. Phytic acid (4).

Some antinutrients and their ambivalent effects are presented in the following Table 1:

Table 1. Ambivalent effects of so-called *antinutrients* in beans

Antinutrient	Ambivalent Effect		Reference
	Deleterious effect	Beneficial effect	
Oligosaccharides: α-galactosides (raffinose, stachyose and verbascose)	Distention and flatulence: Excesive anaerobic fermentation by colonic bacteria, yielding production of hydrogen, CO_2 and traces of methane.	Constituent of dietary fiber: prebiotic effect and increased bifidobacteria colonic population	Martínez-Villaluenga et al., 2008 [13]
	Interaction and reduction in digestion and absorption of nutrients. Changes in small bowel osmotic pressure by increasing fermentable carbohydrates (thus further risk of presenting osmotic diarrhea).	Immune system stimulation: • Microbiota activates the lymphoid tissue associated with gut, by entering through the intestinal epithelial cells or SCFAs produced during prebiotics fermentation influence the immune system by their immunomodulatory and anti-inflammatory properties.	Muzquiz et al., 2012 [9]
Phytic acid (myo-inositol phosphates: IP4, IP5, IP6)	Bivalent mineral (e.g., Cu^{2+}, Zn^{2+}) chelation leading to decreased absorption (risk for nutritional deficiency). Binding with starch through phosphate linkages making it inaccessible to further digestion and absorption. Formation of non-absorbable complexes with proteins and enzymes as α-amylase, pepsin, trypsin and chymotrypsin.	Reduction in bioavailability and therefore toxicity of heavy metals (due to chelation and further absorption inhibition). Antioxidant activity by binding and thereby inactivating ferric ions. Prevention of dystrophic calcifications in soft tissues and kidney stone. Lowering of cholesterol and triglycerides due to decrease dietary absorption	Muzquiz et al., 2012 [9] Doria et al., 2012 [8] Bohn et al., 2008 [14] Valdés et al., 2011[12]

Table 1. (Continued)

Antinutrient	Ambivalent Effect		Reference
	Deleterious effect	Beneficial effect	
		Colon cancer reduction by normalizing abnormal cell proliferation, inducing cell differentiation and apoptosis as well inhibiting angiogenesis.	
Protease inhibitors (Kunitz trypsin inhibitor, Bowman-Birk trypsin/chymotrypsin inhibitors)	Inhibition of digestive enzymes (trypsin and chymotrypsin), by competitive binding with Bowman-Birk protease-inhibitors. Stimulation of pancreatic enzyme secretion, inhibiting intestinal protein digestion.	Inhibition of carcinogenesis, used as chemopreventive and antiproliferative agents in transformed cells. Bowman-Birk inhibitor has been effective preventing human prostate cancer cells, reducing colon tumors.	González de Mejía et al., 2005 [15] Pusztai, et al., 2004 [16]
α-amylase inhibitors (phaseolamin)	Inhibit pancreatic and salivary amylases. Interfere with starch and complex carbohydrate breakdown reducing digestibility.	Treatment of coadjuvant dyslycemia and/or diabetes mellitus (by lowering postprandial blood glucose levels and hence insulinemia).	Muzquiz et al., 2012 [9] González de Mejía et al, 2005 [15] Suarez-Martínez et al, 2016 [17]
Glycoproteins: lectins (phytohemagglutinin (PHA), phytohemagglutinin-L (PHA-L) and leukoagglutinin)	Erythrocytes agglutination. Malnutrition and growth inhibition by binding to the surface of the small intestine epithelial cells and/ or producing immature enterocytes that change the structure and function of the brush of intestinal epithelium	Stimulation of gut function by inducing the release of gut peptide hormones. Tumor growth inhibition (mice non- Hodgkin´s lymphoma) due to competition of nutrients (polyamines). Ameliorating obesity.	Campion et al., 2013 [11] Campion et al., 2009 [18] Zucoloto et al., 1991 [19] González de Mejia et al., 2005 [15]

Antinutrient	Ambivalent Effect		Reference
	Deleterious effect	Beneficial effect	
	membrane interfering with digestion and absorption of nutrients mainly Zn, Fe and proteins. Reduction of the invertase and maltase activity of the intestinal mucosa and with glycose transportation.		Suárez-Martinez et al., 2016 [17]
Saponins	Permeability cell wall alteration and binding to the cells of the small intestine thus, affecting the absorption of nutrients.	Reduced risk of cardiovascular disease and some cancers Reduce cholesterolemia through the formation of insoluble complex with dietary cholesterol (hence decreasing absorption). Inhibition of preneoplastic lesions in mice colon by reduction of azoxymethane.	Lalojo et al., 2004 [20] Muzquiz et al., 2012 [9]

3. Phytochemical Profile

Potential health benefits of beans have been attributed to the presence of alkaloids, polyphenolic compounds, carbohydrates and fiber, oligosaccharides, lectin, trypsin inhibitors, among others. Although, as stated in the prior section, these compounds could be considered as antinutrients (depending on the specific clinical scenario), in this Chapter, we will focus on the beneficial effects that some of these phytochemicals could – and have actually been proven to - provide [21, 22].

3.1. Polyphenolic Compounds

Polyphenols are a large group of compounds that are present in all plants, and therefore many of them are in the diet, but the concentration varies depending on the type of food [23]. Chemically, as seen in Figure 3, the phenolic compounds can be defined as substances that possess an aromatic ring to which one or more hydroxyl - including functional derivatives - groups are attached. According to family structure, polyphenols can be classified as phenolic acids, flavones, flavanones, isoflavones, flavonols, flavanols, anthocyanins and condensed tannins [24].

Phenolics in common beans are found in the seed coats, with lower amounts in the cotyledons. The concentration of these compounds is influenced by growing conditions and genetic factors [25, 26].

Analysis using high performance liquid chromatography-mass spectrometry (HPLC-MS), identified compounds such as anthocyanins, flavanol monomers, and heterogeneous flavanol oligomers up to hexamers. The presence of catechins, delphinidin (6) (Figure 4), cyanidins, and phenolic acids such as gallic (7), vanillic (8), caffeic (9), coumaric (10) and ferulic (11) acids (Figure 4) in the seed coat of common beans have been reported [25]. Phenolic compounds such as anthocyanins, quercetin glycosides and proanthocyanidins (condensed tannins), were isolated and identified in dark red kidney beans [27]. The main differences between white and colored beans were the presence of free kaempferol (5) and derivatives (kaempferol-3-*O*-glucoside (12)) (Figure 4), only in red and black beans [28, 29]. The pelargonidin 3-glucoside (13) (Figure 5) is the main anthocyanin found in this colored beans, its structure is shown in Figure 5. Kaempferol (5) and quercetin (14) (Figure 4) have been reported as the main flavonoids in different market classes of Mexican beans [30].

The most widely studied feature –although not necessarily the most important regarding bioactivity of polyphenolic compunds such as flavonoids and anthocyanins is their significant antioxidant activity, however it is not the only pathway that have been describe to explain its important effects in cardiometabolic regulation [24, 31].

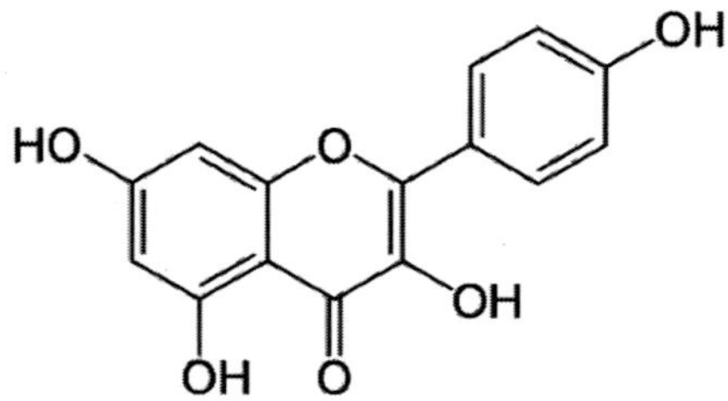

kaempferol (5)

Figure 3. Polyphenolic structure (e.g., kaempferol (5)).

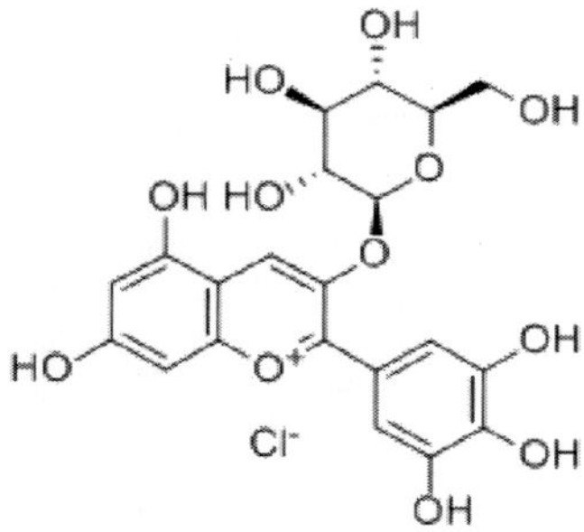

delphinidin (6)

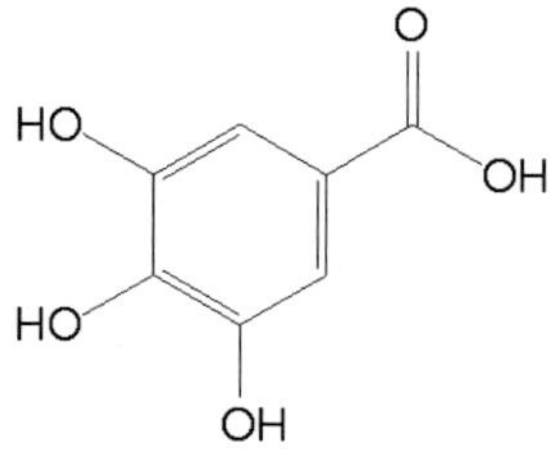

gallic acid (7)

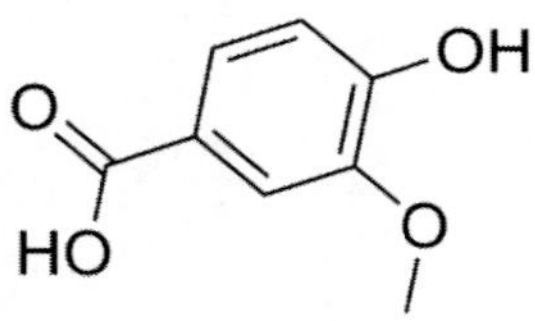

vanillic acid (8)

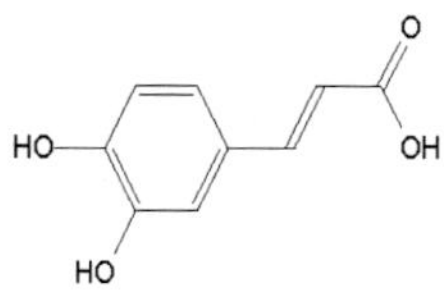

caffeic acid (9)

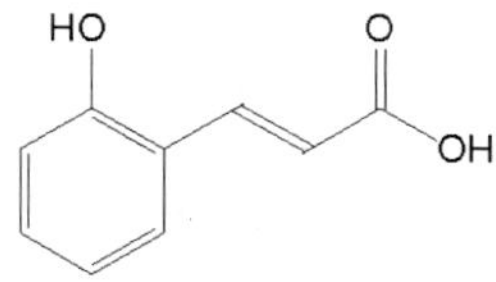

coumaric acid (10)

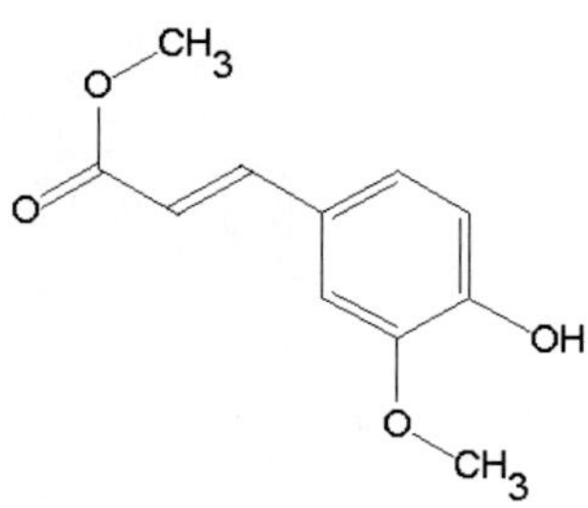

ferulic acid (11)

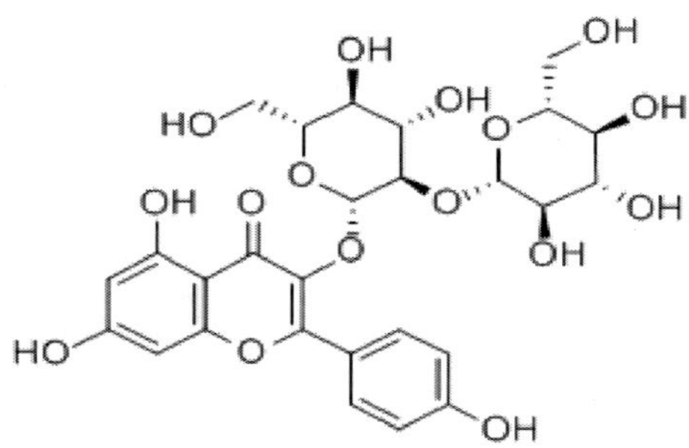

kaempferol-3-*O*-glucoside (12)

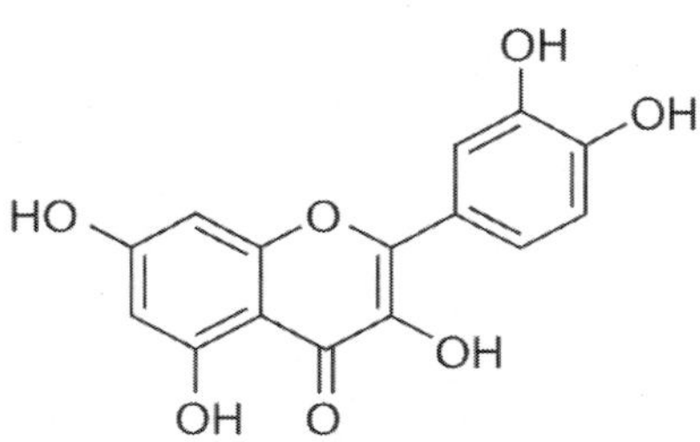

quercetin (14)

Figure 4. Delphinidin (6), gallic acid (7), vanillic acid (8), caffeic acid (9), coumaric acid (10) and ferulic acid (11), kaempferol (5), kaempferol-3-*O*-glucoside (12), and quercetin (14).

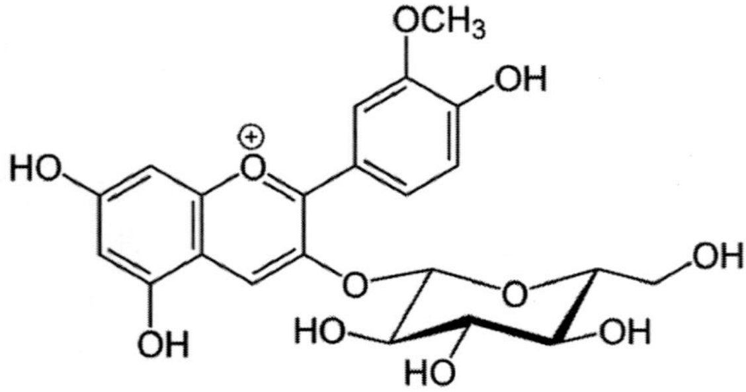

pelargonidin 3-glucoside (13)

Figure 5. Anthocyanin structure (e.g., pelargonidin 3-glucoside (13)).

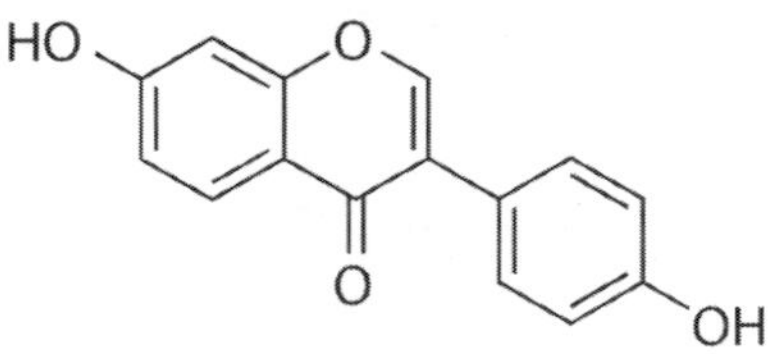

daidzein (15)

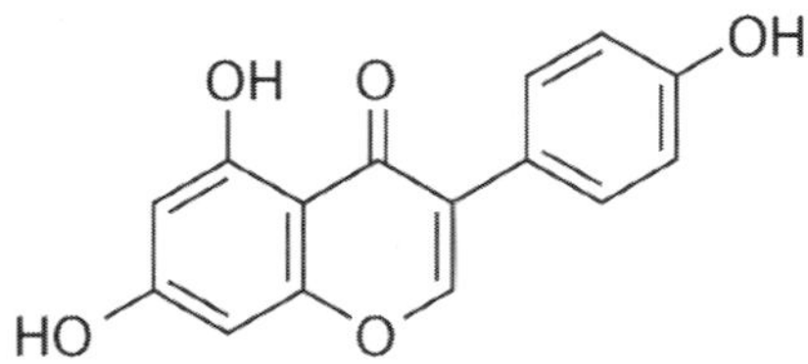

genistein (16)

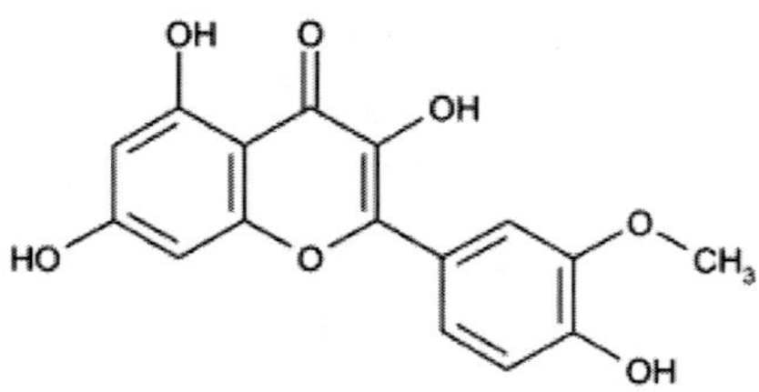

isorhamnetin (17)

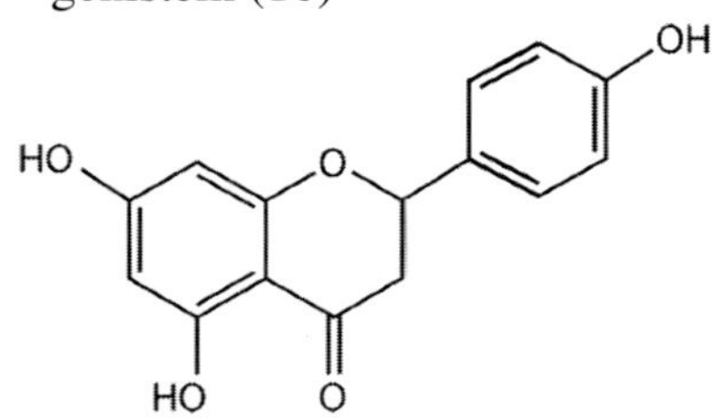

naringenin(18)

Figure 6. Daidzein (15), genistein (16), isorhamnetin (17), and naringenin (18).

Different studies have reported that some polyphenols such as flavone, daidzein (15), genistein (16), isorhamnetin (17) (Figure 6), kaempferol (5), quercetin (14), naringenin (18) (Figure 6), and pelargonidin inhibited the lipopolysaccharide (LPS)-induced NF-kappa-B (NF-κB) activation. In addition, genistein (16), kaempferol (5), quercetin (14), and daidzein (15) also inhibited signal transducer and activator of transcription 1 (STAT-1) activation. The mechanisms by which phenolic compounds inhibit STAT-1 activation are not known, but may be associated with inhibition of phosphorylation of STAT-1 or its up-stream kinase Janus kinase 2 (JAK2).

Some researches have report that genistein (16), kaempferol (5), and quercetin (14) are potent inhibitors of inducible nitric oxide synthase (iNOS) expression and nitric oxide (NO) production, inhibiting both NF-κB and STAT-1 activations [32].

3.2. Fiber

Common beans, like other legumes, also contain significant amounts fiber. In beans, carbohydrates constitute the main fraction of grain legumes, accounting up to 55-65% of the dry matter. Of these, starch and non-starch polysaccharides (dietary fiber) are the major constituents, with smaller but significant amounts of mono-, di- and oligosaccharides (these are discussed in the following sub-heading). Dietary fiber represents 15-48% in different types of common beans [33, 34, 35].

Research has demonstrated that consumption of dietary fiber and resistant starches - both available from dry beans - are associated to specific physiological responses that are of health significance [36]. For example, non-digested carbohydrates (National Drug Code (NDC) system - including resistant starch, soluble and insoluble dietary fiber, together with non-digestible oligosaccharides - are associated with a low glycemic response, low serum cholesterol levels, and a decrease of colon cancer risk. Such effects of NDC may be related to colonic fermentation end products, including short chain fatty acids (SCFA) such as propionic (19) and butyric (20) acids (Figure 7) [37, 38, 39, 40).

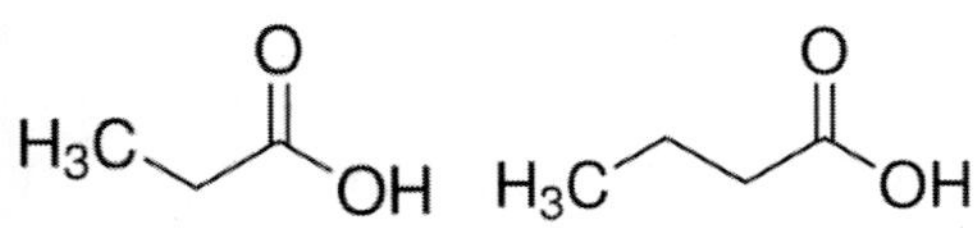

propionic (19) butyric acid (20)

Figure 7. Propionic (19) and butyric acid (20).

3.3. Oligosaccharides

This family of molecules is known as α-galactosides (raffinose family of oligosaccharides, RFO), and derived from sucrose (21) (Figure 8) and have 1-3 α-1,6-linked galactosyl units attached. They are commonly known as raffinose (1 galactosyl unit. 22), stachyose (2 galactosyl units. 23), and verbascose (3 galactosyl units. 24) (Figure 8), and also have been shown to be able to stimulate the growth and activity of beneficial bacteria or prebiotic agent. Also, oligosaccharides affect different gastrointestinal activities and lipid metabolism, to enhance immunity, and to reduce diabetes, obesity and cardiovascular risk. α-Galactosides are not digested in the upper part of the gastrointestinal tract, due to the absence of α-galactosidase among human endogenous enzymes, and are therefore available for bacterial fermentation in the colon to produce a mixture of short-chain fatty acid (SCFA) which may have several beneficial implications for health, such as protective effects against colorectal cancer [13, 41, 42].

The content of total oligosaccharides in different beans ranged from 9 to 30 mg/g, among which stachyose (23) ranged from 4 to 15 mg/g, raffinose (22) content ranged from 3.2 to 63.8 mg/g, and verbascose (24) ranged from 0.24 to 5.1 mg/g [8, 43].

3.4. Lectins

Lectins constitute a heterogeneous group of glycoproteins, often resistant to proteolysis within the gastrointestinal tract, and which characteristically exhibit the ability to agglutinate blood cells thus are often called phytohemagglutinin (PHA) [44].

Lectin consists of five different tetramers formed by two polypeptide chains: leukoagglutinating phytohemagglutinin (L-PHA) and erythro-agglutinating phytohemagglutinin (E-PHA). They consist of five tetrameric lectins designated L4, L3E1, L2E2, L1E3, and E4 based on the number of L and E polypeptide subunits/molecule. Lectin content in legumes is in the range of 5 to 20% w/w [45, 46, 47]. Significant amounts of lectins have been found in *Phaseolus vulgaris* beans [48].

These molecules possess at least one non-catalytic domain that enables them to selectively recognize and binds reversibly to a specific mono- or oligosaccharide present on glycoproteins and glycolipids [49]. This property gives them a diversity of biological functions such as preventing certain cancers, in the activation of certain innate defense mechanisms and may be used as a therapeutic agent for preventing or controlling obesity. In addition, lectins exhibit, immunomodulatory, antifungal, antiviral, and human immunodeficiency virus type 1 (HIV-1) reverse transcriptase inhibitory activities [46, 47, 50-56].

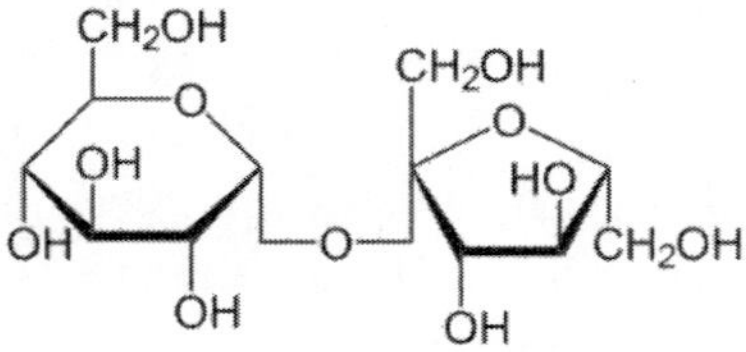

sucrose (21)

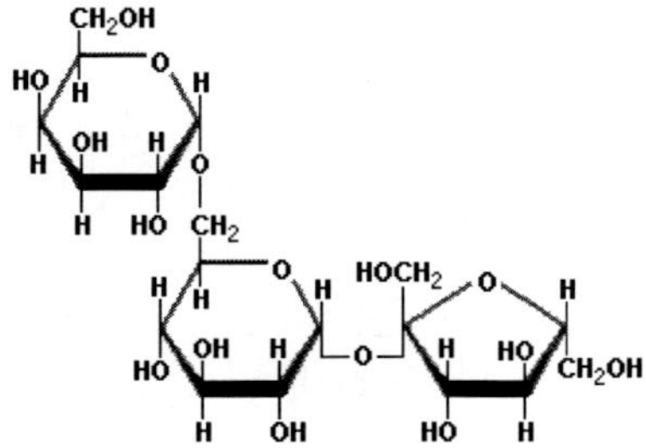

raffinose (22)

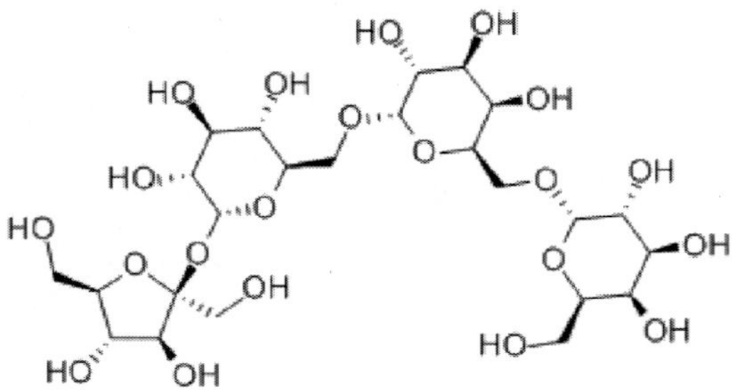

stachyose (23)

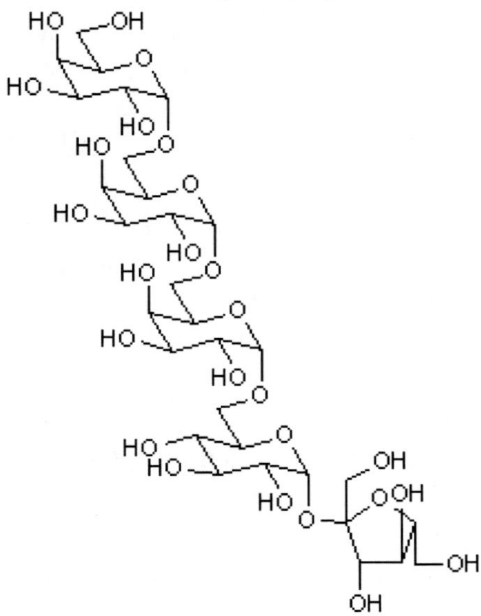

verbascose (24)

Figure 8. Sucrose (21), raffinose (22), stachyose (23), and verbascose (24).

3.5. Amylase Inhibitors

Phaseolus vulgaris (P. vulgaris) has non-nutritive bioactive factors named as starch blockers, which are substances that interferes the rupture of complex carbohydrates that cause a prolonged digestion. These factors are α-amylase inhibitors (α-AI), phytohaemagglutinin (PHA) and arcelins (promoter of seed storage protein) which have been extracted and used in different products commercialized as supplement with different brands such as an α-amylase inhibitor phaseolamin and Phase-2. Among the α-amylase inhibitors, the isoform 1 is the most widely distributed and the one has demonstrated α-amylase inhibitory activity in humans [57, 58].

The inhibitor of α-amylase activity cause weight reduction through energy restriction due to the mobilization of the body's fat. P. vulgaris is also used to reduce body weight through appetite suppression [57, 58, 59].

3.6. Weight-Management Potential

It has been well recognized for many years now that obesity is a major health hazard associated to comorbidities such as cardiovascular disease, type 2 diabetes; musculoskeletal disorders, and certain types of cancer. In spite of its rising epidemiological figures, there is no effective long-term treatment for it: although therapeutic changes in lifestyle, i.e., diet and exercise, certainly have beneficial effects, they tend to fail due to poor compliance; for its side, approved anti-obesity drugs like a neutral fat absorption inhibitor (orlistat. xenical), 5-hydroxytryptamine (serotonin) 3 receptor stimulator (lorcaserin) and a central appetite depressant phentermine/an antiepileptic drug topiramate, are frequently associated to side effects. In view of these drawbacks, a shift towards formerly considered *alternative* therapies such as the use of functional foods - with minimal side effects - is growing.

Some murine model studies exhibited the beneficial effects of *Phaseolus vulgaris* in the treatment of overweight and obesity; thus, *P. vulgaris* is considered as an anti-obesity agent. In 2011, Carai et al., administrated a standardized *P. vulgaris* dry extracts (PVE) at 50 and 500 mg/kg in three 5-day treatment periods followed by three 20 days off treatment periods, resulted in a loss of 20-30% in daily food intake and 40% of body weight at both doses and being dose-dependent [60]. In 2012, Meanwhile Zhu et al., evaluated the incorporation of cooked dry bean into a diet to assess the effect on Sprague-Dawley rats and a diet-induced obesity model in C57B1/6 mice observed that in both animal species, the consumption of bean-diet improved plasma lipid profile and body weight loss [61].

In 2013, Loi et al., treated mice CD1 with a standardized *P. vulgaris* dry extracts (PVE) at 500 and 1000 mg/kg; and then exposed to unlimited access to food (regular pellets, butter cookies, condensed milk beverage and chocolate-flavored beverage). Treatment with PVE resulted in food intake reduction [62].

In 2016, Song et al., study the influence of PVE on obesity in high-fat diet fed mice at 50 mg/kg dose. The results showed that PVE treatment reduced body weight gain as well as the relative weight of visceral white adipose compared to mice fed only with high-fat diet [63].

In 2007, regarding clinical scenarios, trials such as the one of Celleno et al., evaluated a PVE (445 mg) dietary supplement in slightly overweight subjects with a high carbohydrate rich calorie diet. After 30 days of treatment subjects had significant reductions of body weight (4%), fat mass (10%), and waist/hip circumferences (3/1.3%, respectively) compared with the baseline [64]. In 2007, meanwhile Udani et al., conduct a pilot study to determine the effect of the intake of PVE (1000 mg) modifying behavior, exercise and diet. The treatment with PVE reduced weight (3.4%) and waist size (2.2%) significantly from baseline [65].

In 2010, Wu et al., examined a PVE (1000 mg) dietary supplement three times per day on subjects with a body mass index (BMI) 25 - 40 kg/cm^2. After 60 days of treatment subjects had significantly reduction of body weight (1.9 Kg) and waist circumference (1.9 cm) [66].

In 2014, Luzzi et al., evaluated the efficacy of 100 mg of PVE (Beanblock®) on weight control in healthy overweight subjects (body mass index (BMI) 25-30 kg/m^2) during 12 weeks. The supplementation with Beanblock® was associated not only with body weight ~4 kg and ~6 cm of waist circumference reduction but also with decreased in oxidative stress [67].

The anti-obesity action of PVE is associated with various mechanisms one of them relies on α-amylase-inhibiting activity of *P. vulgaris* which promote weight loss interfering with the digestion of complex carbohydrates to simple; decelerating carbohydrate absorption; thus, reducing carbohydrate-derived calorie by influencing the insulin system that could lead to lesser fat accumulation [59, 63-69] and mobilizing fat reserves because of the energy restriction of α-amylase inhibitors [59]. Other PVE anti-obesity mechanism could be due to lectins (hemagglutinins. HAs) which induce reduction in appetite and delay in gastrointestinal transit, probably *via* alterations in the release of cholecystokinin (CCK) and glucagon-like peptide-1 (GLP-1) [59,

60]. Some studies attribute the anti-obesity effect of PVE to the inhibition of fatty acid synthase (FAS) by suppressing appetite, thus, decrease body weight.

Although the aforementioned evidence is quite interesting, more studies with larger samples are indeed needed to draw certain conclusions on the effects of *P. vulgaris* in regards of weight modulation and, moreover, to elucidate its intricate anti-obesity mechanisms.

3.7. Hunger/Satiety Regulation

Given that obesity results from an imbalance between energy intake and expenditure, the regulation of food intake has been a target for treatment for many years; common bean extracts have not been the exception: its anorexigenic effect has certainly been studied, although its mechanism it's not completely understood. Some proposals attribute this effect to a retard in gastric emptying due to the stimulation of cholecystokinin (CCK) release resulting from the phytohaemagglutinin (PHA) binding to the brush-border membrane of the intestine [57, 59, 70].

In 2004, Tormo et al., studied the prolonged oral administration (21 days) to adult Wistar rats of an isolated and purified α-amylase inhibitor (50 mg/kg body weight). The inhibitor has shown reducing feed intake, blood glucose levels and body weight gain [71]. However, in other studies the α-amylase inhibitor didn't show anorexigenic effect in short periods of time. For this results it can be concluded that maybe the anorexigenic effect can be achieved after long exposure to the α-amylase inhibitor [59, 72].

In 2009, Fantini et al., demonstrated reduced postprandial glycaemia and food intake in Wistar rats maintained on a starch-enriched diet due to the administration of PVE at different concentrations (0, 50, 200, and 500 mg/kg) for 10 days. They also evaluated the effect of the pretreatment with a cholecystokinin (CCK) receptor antagonist, lorglumide (0 and 10 mg/kg), this pretreatment blocked the effect on the food intake of PVE, that suggest the possible mechanism of the satiety effect of PVE is mediated by CCK receptors and not only by α-amylase [62].

In 2011, Carai et al., evaluated the effect of multiple cycles of repeated treatments with PVE on food intake and body weight in genetically obese Zucker fa/fa rats. For this purpose, they administered doses of 0, 50 and 500 mg of PVE/kg once a day during 5 days followed by 20 days of no treatment, and repeated these periods three times. The effect of PVE decreasing food intake, body weight and glycaemia was dose-dependent in each treatment phase. Reductions in food intake were of comparable magnitude in each treatment. With this results, they concluded that PVE has potential to be used as pharmacotherapy for obesity and related disorders [73].

In 2010, Maccioni et al., demonstrated that PVE can reduce the intake of a chocolate-flavored beverage. In this study rats were initially trained to lever – press for a chocolate-flavored beverage. After this trained, rats were pretreated with an intragastric administration of 50, 200 and 500 mg of PVE/kg, the results showed a reduction in liver - responding for the chocolate beverage was 15, 35 and 40% respectively [74]. In 2013, Loi et al., also studied the effect of PVE on intake of palatable foods by mice. Mice in different groups, had unlimited access to regular food pellets or limited access (1 hr) to butter cookies, condensed milk and a chocolate flavored beverage. The treatment with PVE, demonstrated a reduction in the intake of regular and palatable food. In these studies, they hypothesized that maybe the satiety effect is due to mechanisms that involved central regulation of appetite [75].

In 2013, Spadafranca et al., used a purified PVE (100 mg) as a supplement in a balanced meal and evaluate plasma glucose, ghrelin (an enzyme produced by stomach lining cells that stimulates appetite) and satiety sensation ratings during 3 hrs after meal consumption. The volunteers were six females and six males (20 – 26 years) with normal weight (BMI 19.7 – 23.5 kg/m^2). The consumption of PVE resulted in lower increments in glucose at 30 min after ingestion compared with the placebo ingestion. Ghrelin is an orexigenic peptide secreted by the stomach and act like a hunger signal, high plasma ghrelin concentration increases food intake. In this study, plasma ghrelin decreased with PVE and placebo consumption, but in the case of placebo the content of ghrelin rebound after 2 h, also demonstrated that PVE induced a higher satiety sensation after 3 hrs [57].

CONCLUSION

Phaseoulus vulgaris L, the common bean, is consumed worldwide due to its nutritional profile, mainly related to protein content and amino acidic recount. However, this legume also contains bioactive substances capable of modulating metabolic pathways related to energy metabolism hence exhibiting a potential role on the treatment of weight control and obesity. Although some evidences in both the preclinical and the clinical scenarios have appointed to beneficial effects including reductions in body weight, abdominal circumference, body composition (fat mass and lean mass), satiety and appetite [67, 73, 76, 77], more robust evidence is needed in order to include Phaseoulus vulgaris – either as a nutraceuticals preparation or a functional food - within the everyday treatment for obesity [58] and, moreover, its associated comorbidities.

REFERENCES

[1] Duke JA, Bigenschutz-Godwin MJ, duCellier J, Duke PAK. *Handbook of Medicinal Herbs*. New York. CRC Press, USA, 2002.

[2] Câmara C, Urrea CA, Schlegel V. Pinto Beans (*Phaseolus vulgaris* L.) as a functional food: implications on human health. *Agriculture* 3(1), 90–111, 2013.

[3] Luna-Vital DA, Mojica L, de Mejía EG, Mendoza S, Loarca-Piña G. Biological potential of protein hydrolysates and peptides from common bean (*Phaseolus vulgaris* L.): A review. *Food Research International* 76(1), 39–50, 2015.

[4] Watson RR, Preedy VR (eds). *Bioactive Food as Dietary Interventions for Liver and Gastrointestinal Disease.* 1st ed, Academic Press, USA, 2012.

[5] Center for New Crops & Plants Product, Prude University. *Phaseolus vulgaris* L. 1998. <https://hort.purdue.edu/newcrop/duke_energy/Phaseolus_vulgaris.html>.

[6] Raatz S. Nutrition value of dry beans. The Bean Institute. Research Nutritionist, USDA Human Nutrition Research Center, Grand Forks, North Dakota, USA, 2016. < http://beaninstitute.com/nutritional-value-of-dry-beans/>.

[7] Romero-Arenas O, Damián HMA, Rivera TJA, Báez SA, Huerta LM, Cabrera HE. The nutritional value of beans (*Phaseolus vulgaris* L.) and its importance for feeding of rural communities in Puebla-Mexico. *Int Res J Biological Sci* 2(8), 59-65, 2013.

[8] Doria E, Campion B, Sparvoli F, Tava A, Nielsen E. Anti-nutrient components and metabolites with health implications in seeds of 10 common bean (*Phaseolus vulgaris* L. and *Phaseolus lunatus* L.) landraces cultivated in southern Italy. *J Food Compos Anal* 26(1–2), 72–80, 2012.

[9] Muzquiz M, Varela A, Burbano C, Cuadrado C, Guillamón E, Pedrosa MM. Bioactive compounds in legumes: Pronutritive and antinutritive actions. Implications for nutrition and health. *Phytochem Rev* 11, 227-244, 2012.

[10] Savelkoul FH, Tamminga S, Leenaars PP, Schering J, Ter Maat DW. The degradation of lectins, phaseolin and trypsin inhibitors during germination of white kidney beans, *Phaseolus vulgaris* L. *Plant Foods Hum Nutr* 45(3), 213-222, 1994.

[11] Campion B, Glahn RP, Tava A, Perrone D, Doria E, Sparvoli F, Cecotti R, Dani V, Nielsen E. Genetic reduction of antinutrients in common bean (*Phaseolus vulgaris* L.) seed, increases nutrients and *in vitro* iron bioavailability without depressing main agronomic traits. *Field Crop Res* 141, 27-37, 2013.

[12] Valdés ST, Coelho CMM, Michelluti DJ, Tramonte VLCG. Association of genotype and preparation methods on the antioxidant activity, and antinutrients in common beans (*Phaseolus vulgaris* L.). *LWT - Food Sci Technol* 44(10), 2104-2111, 2011.

[13] Martínez-Villaluenga C, Frias J, Vidal-Valverde C. Alpha-galactosides: antinutritional factors or functional ingredients? *Crit Rev Food Sci Nutr* 48(4), 301-316, 2008.

[14] Bohn L, Meyer AS, Rasmussen SK. Phytate: Impact on environment and human nutrition. A challenge for molecular breeding. *J Zhejiang Univ Sci B* 9(3), 165-191, 2008.

[15] De Mejía EG, Prisecaru VI. Lectins as bioactive plant proteins: a potential in cancer treatment. *Crit Rev Food Sci Nutr* 45(6), 425–445, 2005.

[16] Pusztai, A., Bardocz S, Martín-Cabrejas MA. The mode of action of ANFs on the gastrointestinal tract and its microflora. In: Muzquiz M, Hill GD, Cuadrado C, Pedrosa MM (eds). *Recent advances of research in antinutritional factors in legume seeds and oilseeds*. pp. 87-100. Wageningen Academic Publishers, The Netherlands, 2004.

[17] Suárez-Martínez SE, Ferriz-Martínez RA, Campos-Vega R, Elton-Puente JE, Carbot KDLT, García-Gasca T. Review. Bean seeds: leading nutraceutical source for human health. *CyTA - J Food* 14(1), 131-137, 2016.

[18] Campion B, Perrone D, Galasso I, Bollini R. Common bean (*Phaseolus vulgaris* L.) lines devoid of major lectin proteins. *Plant Breeding* 128(2), 199–204, 2009.

[19] Zucoloto S, Scaramello AC, Lajolo FM, Muccillo G. Effect of oral phytohaemagglutinin intake on cell adaptation in the epithelium of the small intestine of the rat. *Int J Exp Pathol* 72(1), 41-45, 1991.

[20] Lajolo FM, Genovese MI, Pryme IF, Dale TM. Beneficial (antiproliferative) effects of different substances. In: Muzquiz M, Hill GD, Cuadrado C, Pedrosa MM (eds). *Recent advances of research in antinutritional factors in legume seeds and oilseeds.* pp.123-135. Wageningen Academic Publishers, The Netherlands, 2004.

[21] Beninger CW, Hosfield GL. Antioxidant activity of extracts, condensed tannin fractions, and pure flavonoids from *Phaseolus vulgaris* L. seed coat color genotypes. *J Agric Food Chem* 51(27), 7879-7883.

[22] Espinosa-Alonso LG, Lygin A, Widholm JM, Valverde ME, Paredes-Lopez O. Polyphenols in wild and weedy Mexican common beans (*Phaseolus vulgaris* L.). *J Agric Food Chem* 54(12), 4436-4444, 2006.

[23] Scalbert A, Manach C, Morand C, Rémésy C, Jiménez L. Dietary polyphenols and the prevention of diseases. *Crit Rev Food Sci Nutr* 45(4), 287–306, 2005.

[24] Giada MDLR. Chapter 4. Food phenolic compounds: main classes, sources and their antioxidant power. In: Morales-González JA (ed). *Oxidative Stress Chronic Degener Dis - A Role Antioxidants*. pp. 87-112, 2013, Science, Technology and Medicine open access publisher (INTECH).

[25] Nyau V, Prakash S, Rodrigues J, Farrant J. HPLC-PDA-ESI-MS identification of polyphenolic phytochemicals in different market classes of common beans (*Phaseolus vulgaris* L.). *Int J Biochem Res Rev* 8(4), 1-11, 2015.

[26] Aparicio-Fernandez X, Yousef GG, Loarca-Pina G, De Mejia E, Lila MA. Characterization of polyphenolics in the seed coat of black jamapa bean (*Phaseolus vulgaris* L.). *J Agric Food Chem* 53(11), 4615–4622, 2005.

[27] Boateng J, Verghese M, Walker LT, Ogutu S. Effect of processing on antioxidant contents in selected dry beans (*Phaseolus spp.* L.). *LWT - Food Sci Technol* 41(9), 1541-1547, 2008.

[28] Hu Y, Cheng Z, Heller LI, Krasnoff SB, Glahn RP, Welch RM. Kaempferol in red and pinto bean seed (*Phaseolus vulgaris* L.) coats inhibits iron bioavailability using an *in vitro* digestion/human Caco-2 cell model. *J Agric Food Chem* 54(24), 9254–9261, 2006.

[29] Laparra JM, Glahn RP, Miller DD. Bioaccessibility of phenols in common beans (*Phaseolus vulgaris* L.) and iron (Fe) availability to Caco-2 cells. *J Agric Food Chem* 56(22), 10999-11005, 2008.

[30] Lin LZ, Harnly JM, Pastor-Corrales MS, Luthria DL. The polyphenolic profiles of common bean (*Phaseolus vulgaris* L.). *Food Chem* 107(1), 399-410, 2008.

[31] Gutiérrez-Salmeán G, Ceballos-Reyes G, Ramírez-Sánchez I. Obesity and metabolic syndrome: Future therapeutics based on novel molecular pathways. *Clin Invest Arter* 24(4), 204–211, 2012.

[32] Hämäläinen M, Nieminen R, Vuorela P, Heinonen M, Moilanen E. Anti-inflammatory effects of flavonoids: genistein, kaempferol, quercetin, and daidzein inhibit STAT-1 and NF-kappaB activations, whereas flavone, isorhamnetin, naringenin, and pelargonidin inhibit only NF-kappaB activation along with their inhibitory effect on iNOS expression and NO production in activated macrophages. *Mediators Inflamm* 2007;2007: 45673. doi: 10.1155/2007/45673.

[33] Tosh SM, Yada S. Dietary fibres in pulse seeds and fractions: Characterization, functional attributes, and applications. *Food Research International* 43(2), 450-460, 2010.

[34] Boye J, Zare F, Pletch A. Pulse proteins: Processing, characterization, functional properties and applications in food and feed. *Food Research International* 43(2), 414–31, 2010.

[35] McCrory MA, Hamaker BR, Lovejoy JC, Eichelsdoerfer PE. Pulse consumption, satiety, and weight management. *Adv Nutr An Int Rev J* 1(1), 17–30, 2010.

[36] Granito M, Michel C, Frías J, Champ M, Guerra M. Fermented *Phaseolus vulgaris*: acceptability and intestinal effects. *Eur Food Res Technol* 220(2), 182–186, 2005.

[37] Chung H-J, Liu Q, Pauls KP, Fan MZ, Yada R. *In vitro* starch digestibility, expected glycemic index and some physicochemical properties of starch and flour from common bean (*Phaseolus vulgaris* L.) varieties grown in Canada. *Food Res Int* 41(9), 869-875, 2008.

[38] Osorio-Díaz P, Bello-Pérez L, Agama-Acevedo E, Vargas-Torres, Tovar J, Paredes-López O. *In vitro* digestibility and resistant starch content of some industrialized commercial beans *(Phaseolus vulgaris* L.). *Food Chem* 78(3), 333-337, 2002.

[39] Ovando-Martínez M, Bello-Pérez LA, Whitney K, Osorio-Díaz P, Simsek S. Starch characteristics of bean (Phaseolus vulgaris L.) grown in different localities. *Carbohydr Polym* 85(1), 54-64, 2011.

[40] Mudgil D, Barak S. Composition, properties and health benefits of indigestible carbohydrate polymers as dietary fiber: A review. *Int J Biol Macromol* 61, 1-6, 2013.

[41] Tang Y, Chen Y, Jiang H, Nie D. The role of short-chain fatty acids in orchestrating two types of programmed cell death in colon cancer. 7(2), 235-237, 2011.

[42] Qiang X, YongLie C, QianBing W. Health benefit application of functional oligosaccharides. *Carbohydr Polym* 77(3), 435–441, 2009.

[43] Castilla JC, Ávila AR, Orozco AC, C, Martínez CJ, Ortiz GD. Chapter 7. Biologically active compounds in the common bean (*Phaseolus Vulgaris* L.) and their health benefits. In: Mora-Escobedo R, Berrios JDJ, Gutierrez-Lopez GF (eds). *Seeds as Functional Foods and Nutraceuticals: New Frontiers in Food Science*. pp.127-142. Nova Science Publishers, NY, USA, 2014.

[44] Movafagh A, Ghanati K, Amani D, Mahdavi SM, Hashemi M, Abdolahi DZ, Darvish H, Gholami M, HaghNejad L, Mosammami S, Safari S, Darehgazani R, Rahimi M, Naini NS, Motlagh MG, Zamani M. The structure biology and application of phytohemagglutinin (PHA) in phytomedicine : With special up-to-date references to lectins. *J Paramed Sci 4(Winter 2013)*, 126–141, 2013.

[45] Campos-Vega R, Loarca-Piña G, Oomah BD. REview. Minor components of pulses and their potential impact on human health. *Food Res Int* 43(2), 461-482, 2010.

[46] Zhang J, Shi X, Shi J, Ilic, Xue SJ, Kakuda Y. Biological properties and characterization of lectin from red kidney bean (*Phaseolus Vulgaris*). *Food Rev Int* 25(1), 1-16, 2009.

[47] Nasi A, Picariello G, Ferranti P. Review. Proteomic approaches to study structure, functions and toxicity of legume seeds lectins. Perspectives for the assessment of food quality and safety. *J Proteomics* 72(3), 527–538, 2009.

[48] He S, Simpson BK, Sun H, Ngadi MO, Ma Y, Huang T. *Phaseolus vulgaris* lectins: A systematic review of characteristics and health implications. *Crit Rev Food Sci Nutr* 2015 Oct 19:0.

[49] Lannoo N, Damme EJMV. Lectin domains at the frontiers of plant defense. *Front Plant Sci* 5, 397, 2014.

[50] Fang EF, Pan WL, Wong JH, Chan YS, Ye XJ, Ng TB. A new *Phaseolus vulgaris* lectin induces selective toxicity on human liver carcinoma Hep G2 cells. *Arch Toxicol* 85(12), 1551–1563, 2011.

[51] Lam SK, Ng TB. Isolation and characterization of a French bean hemagglutinin with antitumor, antifungal, and anti-HIV-1 reverse transcriptase activities and an exceptionally high yield. *Phytomedicine* 17(6), 457–462, 2010.

[52] Wong JH, Wan CT, Ng TB. Characterisation of a haemagglutinin from Hokkaido red bean (*Phaseolus vulgaris cv*. Hokkaido red bean). J Sci Food Agric 90(1), 70–77, 2010.

[53] Kosti O, Byrne C, Cocilovo C, Willey SC, Zheng YL. Phytohemagglutinin-induced mitotic index in blood lymphocytes: a potential biomarker for breast cancer risk. *Breast Cancer (Auckl)* 4, 73-83, 2010.

[54] Fang EF, Lin P, Wong JH, Tsao SW, Ng TB. A lectin with anti-HIV-1 reverse transcriptase, antitumor, and nitric oxide inducing activities from seeds of *Phaseolus vulgaris cv*. extralong autumn purple bean.. *J Agric Food Chem* 58(4), 2221–2229, 2010.

[55] Shi Z, An N, Zhao S, Li X, Bao JK, Yue BS. In silico analysis of molecular mechanisms of legume lectin-induced apoptosis in cancer cells. *Cell Prolif* 46(1), 86–96, 2013.

[56] Lam SK, Ng TB. Apoptosis of human breast cancer cells induced by hemagglutinin from *Phaseolus vulgaris cv. Legumi secchi*. *Food Chem* 126(2), 595-602, 2011.

[57] Spadafranca A, Rinelli S, Riva A, Morazzoni P, Magni P, Bertoli S, Battezzati A. *Phaseolus vulgaris* extract affects glycometabolic and appetite control in healthy human subjects. *Br J Nutr* 109(10), 1789-1795, 2012.

[58] Onakpoya I, Aldaas S, Terry R, Ernst E. The efficacy of *Phaseolus vulgaris* as a weight-loss supplement: a systematic review and meta-analysis of randomised clinical trials. *Br J Nutr* 106(2), 196-202, 2011.

[59] Obiro WC, Zhang T, Jiang B. The nutraceutical role of the *Phaseolus vulgaris* alpha-amylase inhibitor. *Br J Nutr* 100(1), 1-12, 2008.

[60] Carai MA, Fantini N, Loi B, Colombo G, Gessa GL, Riva A, Bombardelli E, Morazzoni P. Multiple cycles of repeated treatments with a *Phaseolus vulgaris* dry extract reduce food intake and body weight in obese rats. *Br J Nutr* 106(5), 762-768, 2011.

[61] Zhu Z, Jiang W, Thompson HJ. Edible dry bean consumption (*Phaseolus vulgaris* L.) modulates cardiovascular risk factors and diet-induced obesity in rats and mice. *Br J Nutr* 108(Suppl 1), S66-S73, 2012.

[62] Fantini N, Cabras C, Lobina C, Colombo G, Gessa GL, Riva A, Donzelli F, Morazzoni P, Bombardelli E, Carai MA. Reducing effect of a *Phaseolus vulgaris* dry extract on food intake, body weight, and glycemia in rats. *J Agric Food Chem* 57(19), 9316- 9323, 2009.

[63] Song H, Han W, Yan F, Xu D, Chu Q, Zheng X. Dietary *Phaseolus vulgaris* extract alleviated diet-induced obesity, insulin resistance and hepatic steatosis and alters gut microbiota composition in mice. *J Funct Foods* 20, 236–244, 2016.

[64] Celleno L, Tolaini MV, D'Amore A, Perricone NV., Preuss HG. A dietary supplement containing standardized *Phaseolus vulgaris* extract influences body composition of overweight men and women. *Int J Med Sci* 4(1), 45–52, 2007.

[65] Udani J, Singh BB. Blocking carbohydrate absorption and weight loss: a clinical trial using a proprietary fractionated white bean extract. *Altern Ther Health Med* 13(4), 32–37, 2007.

[66] Wu X, Xu X, Shen J, Perricone NV. Preuss HG. Enhanced weight loss from a dietary supplement containing standardized *Phaseolus vulgaris* extract in overweight men and women. *J Appl Res* 10(2), 73-79, 2010.

[67] Luzzi R, Belcaro G, Hu S, Dugall M, Hosoi M, Ippolito E, Corsi M, Gizzi. Beanblock ® (standardized dry extract of *Phaseolus vulgaris*) in mildly overweight subjects: A pilot study. *Eur Rev Med Pharmacol Sci* 18(20), 3120–3125, 2014.

[68] Barrett ML, Udani JK. A proprietary alpha-amylase inhibitor from white bean (*Phaseolus vulgaris*): A review of clinical studies on weight loss and glycemic control. *Nutr J* 10(1), 24, 2011.

[69] Gamboa-Gómez CI, Rocha-Guzmán NE, Gallegos-Infante A, Moreno-Jiménez MR, Vázquez-Cabral BD, González-Laredo RF. Plants with potential use on obesity and its complications. *EXCLI J* 14, 809–831, 2015.

[70] Balaji M, Ganjayi MS, Kumar GENH, Parim BN, Mopuri R, Dasari S. A review on possible therapeutic targets to contain obesity: The role of phytochemicals. *Obes Res Clin Pract* 10(4), 363-380, 2016.

[71] Tormo MA, Gil-Exojo I, Romero de Tejada A, Campillo JE. Hypoglycaemic and anorexigenic activities of an α-amylase inhibitor from white kidney beans (*Phaseolus vulgaris*) in Wistar rats. *Br J Nutr* 92(5), 785–790, 2004.

[72] Chokshi D. Toxicity studies of Blockal, a dietary supplement containing Phase 2 Starch Neutralizer (Phase 2), a standardized extract of the common white kidney bean (*Phaseolus vulgaris*). *Int J Toxicol* 25(5), 361–371, 2006.

[73] Carai MA, Fantini N, Loi B, Colombo G, Riva A, Morazzoni P. Potential efficacy of preparations derived from *Phaseolus vulgaris* in the control of appetite, energy intake, and carbohydrate metabolism. *Diabetes Metab Syndr Obes* 2, 145–153, 2009.

[74] Maccioni P1, Colombo G, Riva A, Morazzoni P, Bombardelli E, Gessa GL, Carai MA. Reducing effect of a *Phaseolus vulgaris* dry extract on operant self-administration of a chocolate-flavoured beverage in rats. *Br J Nutr* 104(5), 624–628, 2010.

[75] Loi B, Fantini N, Colombo G, Gessa GL, Riva A, Bombardelli E, Morazzoni P, Carai MA. Reducing effect of an extract of *Phaseolus vulgaris* on food intake in mice - focus on highly palatable foods. *Fitoterapia* 85(1), 14–19, 2013.

[76] Celleno L, Tolaini MV, D'Amore A, Perricone NV, Preuss HG. A Dietary supplement containing standardized *Phaseolus vulgaris* extract influences body composition of overweight men and women. *Int J Med Sci* 4(1), 45–52, 2007.

[77] Grube B, Chong WF, Chong PW, Riede L. Weight reduction and maintenance with IQP-PV-101: a 12-week randomized controlled study with a 24-week open label period. *Obesity* 22(3), 645–651, 2014.

In: Nutraceuticals
Editor: Noboru Motohashi
ISBN: 978-1-53611-785-1

Chapter 3

Obtention and Nutraceutical Characterization of an Enzymatic Extract Derived from Rice Bran

Elisa Revilla[1], Consuelo Santa María[1], M. Dolores Herrera[2], Juan Parrado[1,*] and Angélica Castaño[1]

[1]Department of Biochemistry and Molecular Biology,
[2]Department of Pharmacology,
Faculty of Pharmacy, University of Seville, Spain

Abstract

Rice bran is the most abundant by-product obtained from the rice (*Oryza sativa*) milling process. The whole rice grain is rich in bioactive compounds which are found mainly in the bran. This bran contains naturally-occurring antioxidants, mainly γ-oryzanol, tocopherols, tocotrienols and polyphenols. Moreover, proteins from rice bran have a high nutritional value.

Despite having components of biological significance, the nutritional use of rice bran is limited due to its poor water-solubility and to the lipid deterioration that starts soon after bran removal. Using enzymatic

* Corresponding author Email: parrado@us.es.

technology, our group has developed a process that enables a stable, water-soluble enzymatic extract (RBEE) to be obtained from rice bran.

The enzymatic process increases the concentration of minor functional components, making RBEE rich in bioactive compounds. Thus, RBEE has antioxidant and hypocholesterolemic properties, as well as antiproliferative and inmunoactivatory abilities.

Interestingly, in animal models an RBEE-supplemented diet showed beneficial effects on the cardiovascular system. RBEE ameliorates cardio-metabolic risk factors in obese Zucker rats, as well as ameliorating the proinflamatory response and microvascular alterations associated with obesity. Moreover, RBEE also prevents high-fat diet-induced inflammation in adipose tissue of C57BL/6J mice, as well as preventing vascular impairment in ApoE−/− mice.

Keywords: rice bran, enzymatic extract, antioxidant, hypocholesterolemic, functional food, antiproliferative, metabolic syndrome, cardiovascular disease

ABBREVIATIONS

ACh	acetylcholine
COX-2	cycloxigenase-2
DIO	diet-induced-obesity
EDHF	endothelial derived hyperpolarizing factor
eNOS	endothelial nitric oxide synthase
HDL	high-density lipoprotein
HMG-CoA	hydroxy methyl glutaryl coenzyme A
LDL	low-density lipoprotein
IL-1 β	interleukin 1β
IL-6	interleukin 6
iNOS	inducible nitric oxide synthase
IR	insulin resistance
LDL	low density lipoprotein
MGN-3	arabinoxylan
MNC	mononuclear cell
MS	metabolic syndrome
NEFA	non-esterified fatty acids
NF-κB	nuclear factor kappa-B
NO	nitric oxide

NO(x)	nitric oxide metabolites
NOX	NADPH-cytochrome c reductase
PPAR	peroxisome proliferator activated receptor gamma
RB	rice bran
RBEE	enzymatic extract from rice bran
ROS	reactive oxygen species
SMA	small mesenteric arteries
TBARS	thiobarbituric acid-reactive substances
TNF-α	tumor necrosis factor-alpha
UV	ultraviolet

1. Introduction

The role of dietary plant constituents and their derivatives in the prevention and treatment of a wide variety of diseases is long established [1]. Rice (*Oryza sativa*) is the most important staple crop, feeding more than half of the world's population and generating tons of waste such as rice bran (RB), the greatest abundant by-product obtained in the milling process. RB contains many bioactive compounds, being a good source of protein, fat, and antioxidants [2], but is currently under-utilized, in spite of its high potential in the field of functional foods or nutraceuticals. In fact, RB has been shown to have promising health-related benefits in the prevention of different diseases, including cancer, hyperlipidemia, fatty liver, hypercalciuria, kidney stones and heart disease [3, 4].

The health benefit effects of RB could be attributed to its content of bioactive molecules. Chemical studies indicate that RB is a good source of γ-oryzanol and vitamin E (tocotrienols and tocopherols), lipophilic components having a demonstrated antioxidant activity which protect cells from the oxidative damage [5]. In fact, γ-oryzanol is being increasingly focused upon as an ingredient for drugs, nutraceuticals, functional foods as well as cosmetics [6, 7]. Therefore, the preparation of products enriched in the antioxidant components of RB could be of great importance for the treating oxidative stress-associated disorders.

Furthermore, proteins from RB have a high nutritional value [8], with hypoallergenic capacity [9] and they are as effective as soy protein when lowering plasma cholesterol levels [10]. However, the main problem limiting the use of these proteins is their high insolubility due to the aggregation caused by extensive disulfide bonding.

Despite the promising properties of RB, its nutritional use is limited due not only to its poor water-solubility but also to the lipid deterioration that starts soon after bran removal [2, 11]. Due to the presence of lipase, which by decomposing triglycerides promotes rancidity, some of the fat components in RB are quite unstable. In order to avoid these problems and improve the composition in bioactive compounds from RB, different approaches have been tested [12] such as stabilized hexanic RB extract. This is rich in vitamin E and polyphenols, but unsuitable for human consumption due to the use of chemicals in the process [13].

Using enzymatic technology, our group has developed a treatment that involves a biological soft organic matter solubilization, avoiding the use of organic solvents. Our method enables us to obtain an enzymatic extract from rice bran (RBEE) that is stable and water-soluble and also to inactivate the lipase, thus preventing rancidity. Our RBEE showed a greatly increased functionality with applications in different fields [14], thus RBEE has shown a high content in nutraceutical compounds, particularly phytosterols, γ-oryzanol and tocols and an increased content in high nutritional proteins. Accordingly, RBEE showed both *in vivo* and *in vitro*, functional properties such as antioxidant properties [15], hypocholesterolemic activity [16], antiproliferative and inmunoactivatory abilities [17] and beneficial activities against metabolic alterations related to insulin resistance and obesity [18-20], restoring endothelial function and vascular contractility [21- 24].

2. Desing and Obtaining of a Rice Bran Enzymatic Extract with Functional Properties

RB was processed by enzymatic hydrolysis, using an endoprotease mixture (trypsin- and chymotrypsin-like) as hydrolytic agent, in a bioreactor with controlled temperature (60 ºC) and pH (pH 8), using the pH-stat method [25]. The processing of this product follows different steps, including centrifugation, filtration, and concentration, as has been described [26]. The final product is a brown syrup completely soluble in water. One of the main problems of nutritional stability of RB is that the triglycerides break down due to the presence of endogenous lipase, promoting rancidity of the product. The treatment with protease during the enzymatic hydrolysis process totally depleted lipase activity, which maybe the factor responsible for the stabilization of the lipid components of RBEE [14].

2.1. Chemical Characterization

The enzymatic process leads to a drastic change in the chemical composition of the extract. When compared with RB, the protein fraction of RBEE is enriched (Table 1), becoming the main component. This is due to the use of proteases which extract, solubilize and hydrolyze the initial insoluble proteins in brans, reducing the size of original RB proteins to soluble peptides. The enzymatic extract is also enriched with fats that, due to protein interactions, are mainly soluble.

RB is rich in prominent bioactives such as phytosterols, and, interestingly, our RBEE retains major phytosterols described in RB [27], the most abundant phytochemical found being γ-oryzanol (Table 2). This molecule is antitumorogenic, hypocholesterolemic and anti-inflammatory [6, 7], so there is an increasing interest in using it for nutraceuticals and functional foods, as well as for cosmetics purposes.

Rice is also a good source of other lipid molecules such as tocopherols and tocotrienols that are known collectively as vitamin E or tocols. Vitamin E occurs in nature in at least eight different isoforms, four tocopherols and four tocotrienols. The concentration of tocols in RBEE was also analyzed, identifying seven homologues (α-, β-, γ- and δ-tocopherols and α-, γ- and δ-tocotrienols). Of these, γ-tocotrienols were the most abundant, followed by α-tocopherols and α-tocotrienols (Table 3).

Table 1. Chemical characterization of RB and RBEE

%	RB	RBEE
Carbohydrates	51.06 ± 1.89	28.90 ± 2.10**
Fat	22.50 ± 1.90	33.09 ± 2.70**
Protein	16.98 ± 2.00	33.96 ± 4.00**
Ash	9.46 ± 0.25	4.05 ± 0.15**

All data are presented as mean ± S.E.M. of five independent experiments. Statistical significance: **$p < 0.001$ *vs* RB

Table 2. Phytosterol composition

Sterols	RBEE
γ-Oryzanol (mg/g)	8.95 ± 0.8
Brassicasterol (μg/g)	15.0 ± 1.0
2,4-Methylencholesterol (μg/g)	6.9 ± 3.0
Campesterol (μg/g)	871.0 ± 6.9
Campestarol (μg/g)	41.0 ± 3.0
Stigmasterol (μg/g)	504.0 ± 28.0
δ-7-Campesterol (μg/g)	18.0 ± 2.0
Clerosterol (μg/g)	58.0 ± 5.0
β-Sitosterol (μg/g)	1694.0 ± 32.0
Sitostanol (μg/g)	58.0 ± 4.0
δ- Avenasterol (μg/g)	127.0 ± 9.0
δ-5-2,4-Stigmasterol (μg/g)	32.0 ± 2.3
δ-7-Stigmasterol (μg/g)	17.0 ± 2.0
δ-7-Avenasterol (μg/g)	18.0 ± 1.5
Cholesterol (μg/g)	20.0 ± 3.0
Others (μg/g)	73.0 ± 6.2
Total (μg/g)	3233.1 ± 60.0

All data are presented as mean ± S.E.M. of five independent experiments

Table 3. Tocols composition

	RBEE
Tocopherols (μg/g)	
α-tocopherols	38.6 ± 4.0
β-tocopherols	9.9 ± 0.5
γ-tocopherols	20.4 ± 3.0
δ-tocopherols	24.4 ± 4.0
Total	93.4 ± 10
Tocotrienols (μg/g)	
α -tocotrienols	32 ± 2.0
β-tocotrienols	N.D.
γ-tocotrienols	132 ± 9.0
δ-tocotrienols	5.9 ± 0.3
Total	170 ± 15

All data are presented as mean ± S.E.M. of five independent experiments

RBEE components also include polyunsaturated fatty acids (PUFAs), so linoleic acid and linolenic acid constitute 44% of total fatty acid. Finally, RBEE also contains flavonoids (flavonols, 0.62 mg/g; flavanols, 2.90 mg/g) and phenolic acids (20.14 mg/g) [27].

Accordingly, the enzymatic process increases the biovailability of the extract without losing bioactive components.

2.2. Antioxidant Capacity of RBEE

Oxygen-derived free radicals are continuously produced in the cell during cellular metabolism, leading eventually to damage in pivotal biomolecules; so cells have developed several defense systems such as small molecules (tocopherols, ascorbic acid and glutathione) and antioxidant enzymes [28] that help to protect itself against these free radicals. However, oxidative damage is a major contributor to many pathological disorders and nowadays is increasing the interest in finding natural sources of components that can strengthen these cellular antioxidant systems. In this context, trying to identify the bioactive potential of our RBEE, we searched for the antioxidant activity in various experimental approachs.

RBEE showed antioxidant activity against lipid oxidation measured in an emulsion prepared with a fish oil rich in fatty acid very susceptible to oxidation, and also against protein oxidation assayed in rat brain homogenate [29]. Additionally we also tested the antioxidant capacity of RBEE in two cell models: keratinocyte monolayers and reconstructed human epidermis, both irradiated with ultraviolet B (UVB) and found that RBEE decreased lipid peroxidation in both systems [15].

Many components of the extract may contribute to its antioxidant capacity. Tocols (both tocopherols and tocotrienols) act as antioxidants due to their ability to donate phenolic hydrogens (electrons) to lipid radicals [5]. The antioxidant capacity of γ-oryzanol is also widely known and has been attributed to its structure, which includes ferulic acid with radical scavenging activity [30]. Our extract is also rich in polyunsaturated fatty acids (PUFAs) which act as radical scavenging agents contributing to the antioxidant activity. In fact, other natural substances such as *Rosa rubiginosa* oil [31], grape seed oil [32] and soybean-germ oil [33] are used as cosmetics because of their polyunsaturated fatty acid (PUFAs) content, which act as radical scavenging agents. Finally, the antioxidant activity of RBEE may be also related to its relatively high content of sulfur amino acids [29] precursors of two important natural antioxidants: taurine and glutathione (GSH).

Moreover, our extract showed a sun protection factor of 4.8 ± 0.3 [15] that may be related to ferulic acid. It is known that ferulic acid is able to absorb some ultraviolets (UVs) and is therefore a weak sunscreen in itself. When mixed with other antioxidants such as vitamin E, it stabilizes the formulation and acts synergetically to increase photoprotection [34, 35]. This association is particularly effective for reducing thymine dimer mutations known to be associated with skin cancer [36]. Our extract is rich in ferulic and vitamin E, thus we can propose RBEE as a useful natural standardized extract in skin photoprotection with promising applications in the field of dermatology.

2.3. Antiproliferative and Immunoactivatory Ability of RBEE

Cancer is the first or second cause of death in advanced countries, but only 5–10% of all cancer cases can be attributed to genetic defects, whereas the remaining 90–95% have their roots in environment and lifestyle [37]. In fact, it has been reported that more than 30% of human cancers could be prevented by an alternative strategy of appropriate dietary modification [38]. Moreover, anticancer drug therapies are mostly toxic, immunosuppressive, mutagenic, and even carcinogenic [39]. It is necessary, therefore, to search for natural products with chemopreventive properties without deleterious effects.

Interestingly, we found that RBEE induced death in leukemia MOLT-4 cells but not in non-cancerous lymphocytes. Tumoral cells generate great amounts of reactive oxygen species (ROS) that contribute to their capacity to damage and invade normal tissue [40] and a direct correlation can be established between the antiproliferation of cancer cells and antioxidant mechanisms [41]. Thus, we propose that RBEE can exert its antiproliferative effect on MOLT-4 cells through the antioxidant capacity described above.

Additionally, antitumorogenic activity may be due to other properties. It has been reported that isoprenoids, including tocotrienols, inhibit the proliferation of human breast cancer cell lines, suppress the growth of murine B16 melanomas and induce cell-cycle arrest in the G-1 phase and apoptosis in human and murine tumor cells [42]. Finally, because inflammation and oxidative stress are closely linked to tumor promotion, is probably that ferulate esters, with strong anti-inflammatory and anti-oxidative activities act as anti-tumor promoters [43].

Our RBEE also showed immunoactivatory effect on N13 microglia cells [17]. Phagocytic cells, comprised of neutrophils and monocytes/macrophages including microglia in the central nervous system (CNS), play a key role in the innate immune response to infection. Ghoneum and Matsuura, demonstrated that MGN-3, a modified arabinoxylan from RB, is a potent inducer of phagocytic function by macrophage [44] and it may explain the stimulation of N13 cells induced by RBEE.

In conclusion, the beneficial properties of RBEE may not only be due to its naturally-occurring antioxidant property but also to its antitumorogenic and immunostimulatory capacity.

2.4. Beneficial Effects of RBEE on Risk Features Associated to Metabolic Syndrome

Given the promising properties of the RBEE, we studied its potential for preventing chronic diseases that are a major concern in modern societies. In this context, pathologies such as metabolic syndrome (MS) are becoming an important worldwide health problem [45]. MS has been described as a combination of several clinically specific risk features including obesity (central adiposity), dyslipidemia, insulin resistance, glucose intolerance, hypertension and non-alcoholic fatty liver disease. In fact, the clustering of these risk factors is related to an increased risk of cardiovascular diseases and diabetes [46, 47]. The high morbidity of MS can be partly attributed to modern dietary patterns; diets rich in fats and sugars, the main culprits that lead to MS symptoms [48]. Although insulin and other pharmacological strategies are able to control many aspects of diabetes, they inadequately prevent cardiovascular complications associated with metabolic syndrome [47]. In this scenario, it has been established that diet and physical activity are the first choice for improving or alleviating MS symptoms [49, 50]. Nowadays there is an increasing interest in the investigation of food components that may have an effect on MS features in order to facilitate dietary-based therapies. Interestingly, our RBEE has been shown to have a positive effect on MS-related diseases such as dyslipemia, insulin resistance and obesity [18, 19, 20].

2.4.1. RBEE Attenuates Dyslipemia

RB is known to have hypolipidemic effects such as reducing total plasma cholesterol. This has been attributed primarily to phytosterols, tocols, γ-oryzanol and triterpene alcohol [51, 52, 53]. The hypocholesterolemic effect may be related to interference in cholesterol metabolism by some major constituents of RB [54-59] but the antioxidant function also plays a central role [50, 60, 61]. In fact, RB oil has a demonstrated hypocholesterolemic effect both in animal models and in humans [62 - 65]. This effect is mechanistically related to a strong antioxidant activity. Interestingly, a cholesterol-lowering effect of aqueous enzymatic extracts has recently been described by our group [16] and others [66]. Both enzymatic extracts, enriched with functional components, showed strong antioxidant properties *in vitro* [29, 66]. Thus, the antioxidant property, together with its content in γ-oryzanol, phytosterols and tocols may explain the hypocholesterolemic effect of the RBEE.

In order to gain greater knowledge of the metabolic benefits of RBEE, we extended our study to animal models. Obese Zucker rats are an appropriate model for studying the effect of dietary components on factors associated with metabolic disturbances in overweight individuals. These rats are obese, normoglycemic, insulin-resistant, hyperinsulinemic, hypertriglyceridemic, and hypercholesterolemic. As expected, obese Zucker rats fed on an RBEE-supplemented diet clearly improved the pathogenesis of MS by attenuating dyslipidemia (decreasing circulating levels of triglycerides and total cholesterol, yet increasing high-density lipoprotein (HDL)-cholesterol without altering non-esterified fatty acids (NEFA), hypertension and insulin resistance, as well as by restoring obesity-associated hypoadiponectinemia (Table 4) [18].

The lipid-lowering action of our RBEE has been attributed mainly to the phytosterol and γ-oryzanol content. The efficacy of dietary plant sterols in reducing cholesterol levels has led to the introduction of plant sterol esters as food additives as an aid to reducing low-density lipoprotein (LDL)-cholesterol blood levels. The major sterol in RBEE is β-sitosterol which is highly effective in competing with cholesterol for incorporating in mixed micelles. The structural difference between lateral chains of phytosterols and cholesterol is the factor responsible for this particular effect. Furthermore, the lipid-lowering action may be related to different mechanisms such as increasing the fecal excretion of neutral sterols [67] or interfering with cholesterol absorption by inhibiting esterification of free cholesterol by the acetyl-coenzyme A acetyltransferases (ACAT) and increasing the activity and expression of the ATP-binding cassette transporters (ABCG5 and ABCG8) that accelerate cholesterol flow from the cells to the intestinal lumen [68].

Table 4. Biochemical analysis after chronic treatment with RBEE.

	LC	L1	L5	OC	O1	O5
Serum						
TC (mmol/L)	2.35 ± 0.10^{a}	2.4 ± 0.2^{a}	2.59 ± 0.06^{a}	6.0 ± 0.3^{b}	5.4 ± 0.2^{c}	5.0 ± 0.7^{d}
HDL-C (mmol/L)	0.88 ± 0.07^{a}	0.95 ± 0.11^{a}	0.91 ± 0.13^{a}	2.4 ± 0.3^{b}	2.9 ± 0.2^{c}	3.2 ± 0.3^{d}
TC/HDL-C	2.7 ± 0.2^{a}	2.7 ± 0.2^{a}	3.0 ± 0.3^{a}	3.2 ± 0.8^{b}	2.03 ± 0.13^{c}	1.7 ± 0.2^{c}
TG (mmol/L)	0.98 ± 0.15^{a}	0.66 ± 0.08^{a}	0.66 ± 0.07^{a}	4.6 ± 0.6^{b}	4.0 ± 0.2^{c}	3.30 ± 0.15^{d}
NEFA (mmol/L)	0.49 ± 0.04^{a}	0.45 ± 0.14^{a}	0.47 ± 0.04^{a}	0.94 ± 0.10^{b}	0.91 ± 0.03^{b}	0.99 ± 0.11^{b}
Glucose (mmol/L)	6.6 ± 0.6^{a}	5.2 ± 0.6^{b}	5.7 ± 0.3^{a}	8.7 ± 1.0^{c}	9.4 ± 0.5^{c}	9.0 ± 1.0^{c}
Insulin (ng/mL)	0.48 ± 0.12^{a}	0.42 ± 0.11^{a}	0.48 ± 0.08^{a}	4.5 ± 0.6^{b}	4.1 ± 0.5^{c}	2.6 ± 0.6^{d}
HOMA-IR	2.6 ± 0.5^{a}	3.8 ± 0.9^{a}	3.0 ± 0.4^{a}	46 ± 7^{b}	37 ± 4^{b}	22 ± 6^{c}
ALT	74.8 ± 0.5^{a}	73.1 ± 1.0^{a}	67.3 ± 0.8^{a}	90 ± 4^{b}	87 ± 2^{b}	93 ± 6^{b}
AST	141 ± 6^{a}	136 ± 3^{a}	131 ± 2^{a}	126 ± 9^{a}	124 ± 6^{a}	120 ± 8^{a}
Liver						
Total lipids (mg)	76 ± 2^{a}	81 ± 3^{a}	92.6 ± 0.9^{b}	102 ± 4^{c}	99 ± 3^{c}	102 ± 3^{c}
TG (mg/g)	24.8 ± 1.4^{a}	23 ± 3^{a}	38 ± 2^{b}	31.9 ± 0.8^{c}	35 ± 2^{c}	19.17 ± 0.04^{d}
TC (mg/g)	11.0 ± 0.2^{a}	29 ± 2^{b}	30 ± 3^{b}	9.6 ± 0.8^{a}	9 ± 2^{a}	20 ± 2^{c}

Mean ± SEM (n = 7). Values in a row without a common superscript letter differ significantly ($P < 0.05$)

LC, lean controls fed SD; L1, lean fed 1% RBEE-supplemented diet; L5, lean fed 5% RBEE-supplemented diet; OC, obese controls fed SD; 01, obese fed 1% RBEE-supplemented diet; 05, obese fed 5% RBEE-supplemented diet

TB: total cholesterol; HDL-C: high density lipoprotein-cholesterol; TG: triglycerides; NEFA: non-esterified fatty acids; HOMA-IR: homeostatic model assessment-insulin resistance γ-Oryzanol may contribute to the cholesterol-lowering effect of RBEE through the antioxidant activity of its ferulic component. In fact, we have also described that the ferulic acid moiety of γ-oryzanol is the main factor in ameliorating atherosclerosis-related oxidative stress and inflammation in ApoE-/- mice [69]. However, γ-oryzanol has greater effect than ferulic acid on lowering non-HDL-cholesterol plasma levels and on raising plasma HDL-cholesterol, possibly through a greater increase in the fecal excretion of cholesterol and its metabolites [62]. Thus, both γ-oryzanol and ferulic acid may exert anti-atherogenic properties, but through different mechanisms. Additionally triterpene alcohols from γ-oryzanol present a hypocloheste-rolemic activity on themselves [70].

RBEE is also rich in tocotrienols that, as well as its antioxidant property, also lowers serum cholesterol [71] by inhibiting the regulatory enzyme hydroxymethylglutaryl-CoA reductase (HMG-CoA reductase). However, tocotrienols may be converted into tocopherols *in vivo* and α-tocopherol opposes the effect of tocotrienols on the activity of HMG-CoA reductase [72]. Thus, the tocopherols/tocotrienols ratio is of great importance and must be simultaneously equilibrated in order to supplement diets with nutraceutics.

Finally, a lipid-lowering action has also been attributed to the potential hypocholesterolemic and antiatherogenic capacity of proteins from RB [73, 74], since the solubility and bioactivity of these proteins is notably enhanced in RBEE. The beneficial effect may be related to the high concentration of L-arginine in the protein fraction of RBEE (12.7%) [14, 16] because L-arginine dietary supplementation prevents the development of atherosclerosis, probably by converting it into nitric oxide (•NO), which has a variety of beneficial effects on the cardiovascular system [75].

2.4.2. RBEE Attenuates Insulin-Resistance

Insulin resistance (IR), a defining feature of type 2 diabetes, is a state in which physiological concentrations of insulin produce a less than normal response, thereby impairing the capacity of insulin targets to address the metabolic needs of the body. IR is also one of the cardio-metabolic risk factors that characterize MS and it is directly related to increased morbidity and mortality due to cardiovascular and cerebrovascular diseases or kidney and liver dysfunction and failure [76, 77, 78]. This health problem has led to heightened interest in seeking natural and safe compounds to maintain optimal health. In this regard, RB is a good candidate to bear in mind.

Qureshi and coworkers demonstrated that fractions from stabilized RB extract rich in tocopherols/tocotrienols can effectively control blood glucose (blood sugar) levels and IR in diabetic humans [4, 72], while RB oil has been shown to have hypoglycemic activities in diabetic-induced rats [79, 80, 81]. Accordingly, chronic administration of our enzymatic extract, enriched in bioactive compounds present in RB, was found to ameliorate IR in obese Zucker rats [18]. Control of IR and glycemia may be due to the synergistic effect of several bioactive components, mainly tocols and γ-oryzanol, this latter having a potent antioxidant activity that enables the amelioration of diabetes complications such as glycation, glycoxidation and hyperlipemia, as well as exerting indirect effects on glucose absorption, utilization or excretion [4, 72, 80]. Proteins derived from the enzymatic treatment of RB might also be involved in the beneficial effect of RBEE in glucose and insulin metabolism, since these proteins may attenuate formation of advanced glycosylation end products which increase under a diabetic state [4].

Furthermore, adiponectin is a widely recognized insulin sensitizer with specific functions in target tissues related to glucose metabolism and insulin response such as liver, pancreatic β-cells, skeletal muscle or adipose tissue. It seems that while low levels are linked to IR and MS, supplied exogenously or overexpressed as a transgene, adiponectin suffices to promote insulin action and ameliorates IR [82]. Obese Zucker rats are characterized by low serum adiponectin level that may be behind the IR that accompanies the general metabolic alterations in this animal model. Interestingly, chronic RBEE administration restored the adiponectin levels, thus providing protection against the IR which is linked to MS pathogenesis [18].

2.4.3. Positive Effect of RBEE on Obesity

Nowadays it is widely accepted that obesity is characterized by a chronic and systemic low-grade inflammation in adipose tissue. In fact, adipose tissue is no longer considered to be an inert tissue functioning solely as an energy store but also as an endocrine organ that secretes a number of bioactive peptides collectively named adipokines which are relevant at the interface between the immune and the metabolic systems. Among them, adiponectin, which is lower in the serum of patients with visceral obesity and states of IR such as type 2 diabetes [83], is known to have anti-inflammatory effects [84]. Although there is no doubt that in cases of obesity, pro-inflammatory pathways are activated in the adipose tissue itself, the adipose tissue of obese individuals also contains a large number of macrophages, which are an additional source of soluble mediators in the adipose tissue [84]. In fact, inflammation in adipose tissue is partially due to an influx of macrophages that secrete pro-inflamatory factors like tumor necrosis factor (TNF)–α, interleukin (IL)-6, IL-1 beta (IL-1 β) and inducible nitric oxide synthase (iNOS), factors like tumor necrosis factor, interleukin (IL)-6, and inducible nitric oxide synthase (iNOS). Accordingly, in obesity there is a remarkable shift in the pool of tissue macrophages from the alternatively activated M2 type macrophage to the classically activated M1 type macrophage, changing the secretion of cytokines from predominantly anti-inflammatory (M2) to pro-inflamatory (M1) [85].

Taking into account that inflammation and oxidative stress are involved in the spiraling vicious inflammatory cycle [86] and that our RBEE is rich in bioactive compounds with antioxidant activity, RBEE emerges as a good candidate for protecting against the low-grade inflammation linked to obesity. In fact, we found beneficial effects on obese animals through two approaches: genetic and diet-induced obesity. Obese Zucker rats (Zucker diabetic fatty (ZDF) rats) are the best known and most widely used animal model of genetic obesity. They have a point mutation resulting in dysfunctional leptin receptors that makes them leptin-insensitive. Circulatory leptin is an adipokine released by adipose tissue in proportion to the amount of lipids stored and acts on the leptin receptors in the brain, determining a decrease in food intake and an increase in energy expenditure. Therefore, obese Zucker rats develop severe obesity associated with hyperphagia, defective non-shivering thermogenesis and preferential deposition of energy in adipose tissue and they become noticeably obese between the third and the fifth week of life [87].

In terms of the proinflamatory state associated with obesity, obese Zucker rats show overproduction of TNF-α, IL-6, IL-1 β, and inducible nitric oxide synthase (iNOS) in visceral adipose tissue, something that was ameliorated by RBEE supplementation (Figure 1). An RBEE-supplemented diet also improved the unbalanced serum levels of nitric oxide metabolites (NO(x)), iNOS induction biomarkers, in obese rats [18]. This indicates the positive role of RBEE on systemic inflammation which is a key mechanism in the pathogenesis of MS features [46].

In vivo and *in vitro* studies have reported that γ-oryzanol in RB induces anti-inflammatory effects by down-regulating of the inflammatory transcription factor, nuclear factor-kB (NF-κB), which in turn decreases the expression of inflammatory enzymes such as COX-2 and iNOS, and proinflamatory cytokines such as IL-1 β, IL-6, and TNF-α [6]. However, we must not forget that tocotrienols, the main bioactive compound in RBEE, have also been shown to possess anti-inflammatory effects also mediated by inhibiting the NF-κB activation pathway [88, 89, 90].

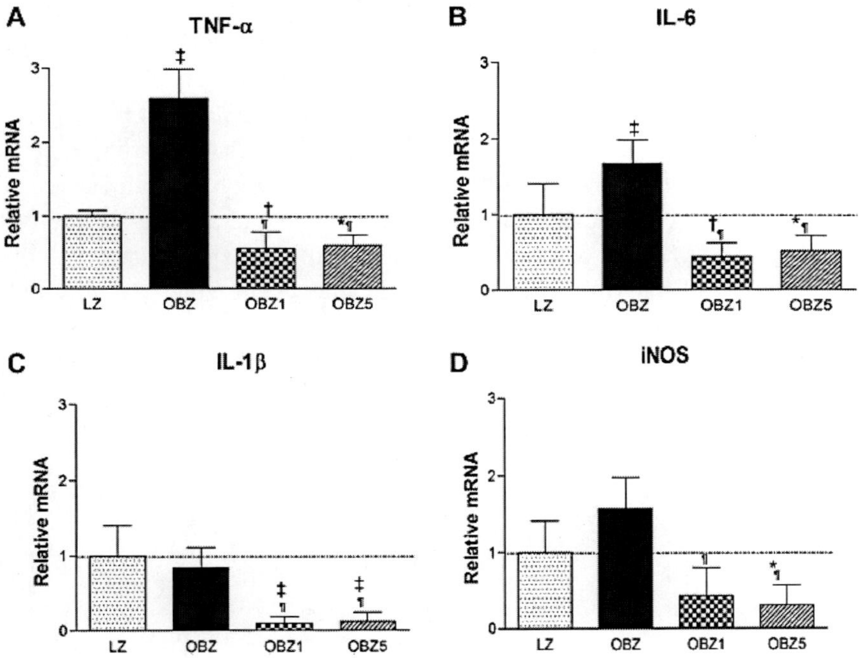

Figure 1. RBEE effect on gene expression of proinflammatory factors. TNF-α (A), IL-6 (B), IL-1 (C) and iNOS (D) in visceral abdominal adipose tissue from lean (LZ) and obese Zucker (OBZ) rats determined using real-time PCR. Experimental groups: LZ, lean control; OBZ, obese control; OBZ1, obese rats fed 1% RBEE-supplemented diet; OBZ5, obese rats fed 5% RBEE-supplemented diet. Data are representative of six to seven rats/treatment group and are expressed as mean ± SEM. $^{*}P < 0.05$; $^{\dagger}P < 0.01$; $^{\ddagger}P < 0.001$ represent a significant differences respect LZ sample using one-way ANOVA with a Tukey's Multiple Comparison Test. P < 0.001 of OBZ1 or OBZ5 with respect to OBZ.

As well as the positive effect found in obese rats, an RBEE-supplemented diet also ameliorated morphological and functional alterations of adipose tissue in DIO (diet-induced-obesity) mice fed on a high-fat-diet [19] that is also a good model for studying obesity. Thus consumption of Western diets, high in sugar and saturated fat, is a crucial contributor to the alarming incidence of obesity and its associated morbidities. RBEE administration in DIO mice ameliorated the obesity-related imbalance in the profile of macrophage phenotypes. While anti-inflammatory M2 macrophages reside in white adipose tissue of lean mice, obese adipose tissue predominantly contains M1 macrophages, a prominent source of pro-inflammatory cytokines such as TNF-α and IL-6 [93]. RBEE treatment decreased the number of macrophage crowns in adipose tissue and restored biomarkers associated with macrophage polarization (i.e., Emr1, Itgax/MRC1 ratio, adiponectin and PPARγ) to levels of lean control mice [19]. This effect can be accomplished by modulating serum adiponectin, known to promote macrophage polarization towards the anti-inflammatory M2 phenotype [94] and to enhance the secretion of the anti-inflammatory cytokine IL-10 [95]. Thus the low levels of adiponectin may underline the M1 classically activated macrophages/M2 alternatively activated macrophages (M1/M2) polarization in obesity. In our experiments, both obese Zucker rats and DIO mice show a hypoadiponectinemia that was restored by RBEE, an effect probably due to γ-oryzanol, given its ability to restore adiponectin levels in obese mice [96]. Furthermore, it is also described that oryzanol upregulated the expression of PPARγ [97], a key molecule in the adiponectin signal transduction pathways [82].

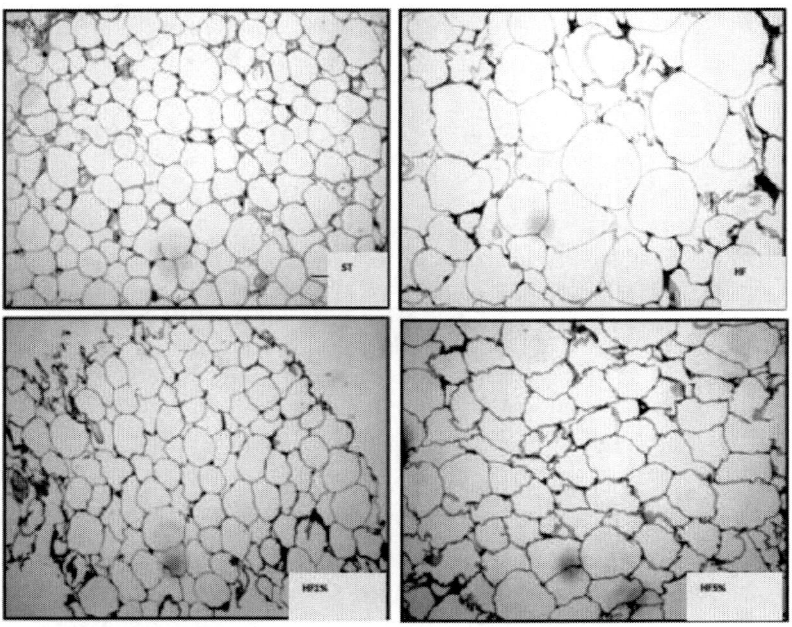

Figure 2. Histology of epididymal white adipose tissue. ST, mice fed standard diet; HF, mice fed high-fat diet; HF1 %, mice fed 1 % RBEE-supplemented high-fat diet; HF5 %, mice fed 5 % RBEE-supplemented high-fat diet.

In addition to ameliorating inflammatory biomarkers in adipose tissue, RBEE also induced a marked shift in adipocyte size distribution toward non-obese animals distribution in both animal models (Figure 2) [20, 19]. Adipose tissue function depends on the adipocyte size and the increase in adipocytes size has been proposed as a predictor of IR development [91, 92].

Summarizing, RBEE-supplemented diet attenuated dyslipidemia, IR and morphological and functional alterations of adipose tissue in obesity animals. Thus, RBEE may be considered as an alternative nutritional complement against MS and its complications.

2.5. Beneficial Effects of RBEE on Cardiovascular System

Recently, interest has emerged in nutritional strategies for preventing and treating cardiovascular diseases [98]. Supplemented diets have the ability to change the structure, composition and function of the arteries, reducing the risk of developing atherosclerosis and thus reduce mortality due to cardiovascular diseases. RB is rich in γ-oryzanol, phytosterols, tocols and ferulic acid, which are known for their interesting lipid reduction, antioxidant and anti-inflammatory activity [2, 6]. RB, therefore, has a great potential both for preventing, and as a therapy for, several chronic human diseases, including allergy, cancer, diabetes, infections, and cardiovascular disease [99]. In fact, the RBEE developed by us has shown its ability to reduce hypertension, restore vascular function in resistance arteries and aorta and reduce oxidative stress in a rat model of metabolic syndrome [18, 20, 21, 22], as well as reducing the plaque burden, it ameliorates atherosclerosis-related oxidative stress and inflammation and has a positive effect on vascular remodeling in ApoE-/- mice [23, 24, 69].

2.5.1. RBEE Has Positive Effects on Hypertension

Obesity is a well-established risk factor for the development of hypertension, since there is a strong correlation between overweight and hypertension [100]. Obesity-related hypertension is associated with both a decrease in the adiponectin concentration and the development of IR, which are in turn related [101]. As discussed above, administering RBEE had a positive concentration-dependent effect on IR and adiponectin levels [20]. Similarly, RBEE had a positive concentration-dependent effect on systolic blood pressure (Figure 3) [18]. There are several studies that confirm the capacity of RB to reduce blood pressure in genetic models of hypertensive rats, ferulic acid being the main factor responsible for this action [102, 103]. Furthermore, a single administration of ferulic acid to spontaneously hypertensive rats induced an attenuation of blood pressure by inhibiting the plasmatic activity of angiotensin-1-converting enzyme activity [104]. The effect of RBEE on vasoconstriction, together with its direct effects on vascular endothelium, might be involved in the attenuation of blood pressure levels previously evidenced in obese Zucker rats treated with this rice bran extract [18, 21].

2.5.2. RBEE Restores Endothelial Function and Vascular Contractility

One of the most characteristic vascular alterations in MS is endothelial dysfunction. This seems to involve a reduction in the amount of the available endothelium-derived NO within the vasculature. Indeed, patients with MS secondary to central obesity show impaired forearm vasodilator response to acetylcholine (ACh) [105]. Considering the beneficial effect of a diet enriched with our RBEE on cardio-metabolic parameters developed in obese rats [18], we studied the capacity of an RBEE-supplemented diet to modify vascular dysfunction in obese Zucker rats, trying to identify the main pathways that could be involved in RBEE's bioactivity.

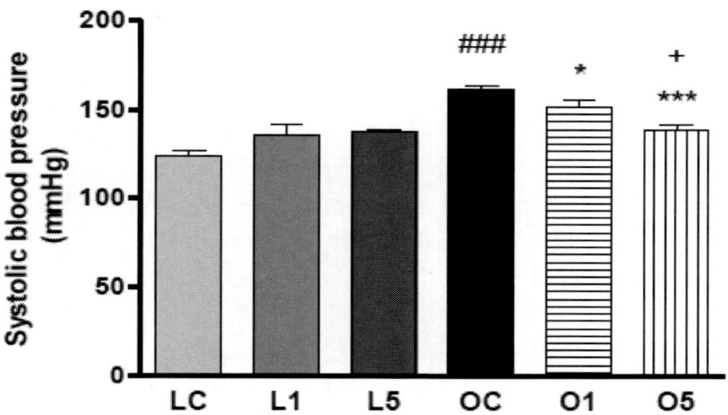

Figure 3. Effect of RBEE treatment on systolic blood pressure.

Final values of systolic blood pressure after 20 weeks of treatment with either standard diet (SD) or rice bran enzymatic extract (RBEE)-supplemented diet. LC lean controls fed SD, L1 lean fed 1 % RBEE-supplemented diet, L5 lean fed 5 % RBEE-supplemented diet, OC obese controls fed SD, O1 obese fed 1 % RBEE-supplemented diet, O5 obese fed 5 % RBEE-supplemented diet. Data are mean ± SEM (n = 7). $^{###}P < 0.001$ versus LC; $^{*}P < 0.05$, $^{***}P < 0.001$ versus OC; $^{+}P < 0.05$ versus O1.

We found that an RBEE-supplemented diet restored the endothelial dysfunction developed by obese Zucker rats [21]. Such a diet upregulated the post-transcriptional activation of eNOS and hence increased endothelial NO production, which is the main mediator of vasodilatation in conductance arteries such as aorta. Obese Zucker rats also show vascular hyperreactivity, evidenced by an increased vascular tone that has been associated with an increased myogenic activation [106], an elevated expression and activity of serotonin [107], and endothelin receptors [108], as well as an increase in sympathetic nervous system activity [109]. RBEE treatment ameliorated hypercontractility to phenylephrine, reaching a vasoconstriction profile similar to lean rats. This response had an important endothelium-dependent component and revealed a different grade of participation of nitric oxide synthase (NOS) isoforms. The up-regulation of endothelial nitric oxide synthase (eNOS) might be involved in the attenuation of vascular vasoconstriction to phenylephrine in intact aortic segments. In addition, selective inhibition of iNOS revealed an important contribution of this isoform in the aortic hyperreactivity of obese Zucker rats.

The excessive NO production from iNOS has been shown to reduce insulin-mediated glucose uptake and induce cellular stress and pancreatic β-cell death in obese animals [110]. Our studies confirmed that obesity is characterized by iNOS overexpression in the vasculature and while obese animals showed augmented values of iNOS aortic protein expression and mRNA levels, these parameters were significantly restored in aortas in RBEE-treated animals. This finding suggests the potential action of RBEE on obesity-related vascular inflammation, which will be discussed later.

Vascular oxidative stress plays a key role in the vascular impairment associated with MS. In general, treatment of obese Zucker rats with antioxidants has improved vasodilator responses to NO-dependent stimuli in isolated microvessels and using *in situ* preparations [111]. In this regard, when evaluating the antioxidant effects of RBEE in vascular tissue, a reduction in RBEE-treated aortas in the expression of the nicotinamide adenine dinucleotide phosphate (NADPH) oxidase subunits NOX-1 and p22phox proteins was found. The concentration of these molecules increased greatly in obese animals, contributing to vascular dysfunction and partially to hypertension. Vascular ROS generation may be the upstream target of RBEE followed by the improvement of vascular reactivity and inflammatory biomarkers. Using animal models with genetic disruption of subunits of the enzyme, several studies support the important role of NADPH oxidase-derived ROS in hypertension and atherosclerosis [112, 113].

Vascular function impairment in MS also implies proinflamatory mediators. Interestingly, RBEE attenuated vascular inflammation by not only reducing aortic iNOS but also by TNF-α expression. Therefore, we can conclude that an RBEE-supplemented diet ameliorates obesity-related vascular impairment by restoring endothelial dysfunction and vascular hyperreactivity *via* a counteraction of iNOS and TNF-α involvement, probably in association with a notable reduction in vascular oxidative stress (Figure 4). Altogether, the beneficial effect of RBEE on vascular alterations linked to MS seems to be a consequence of a reduction in vascular, adipose and plasmatic proinflamatory and pro-oxidant biomarkers together with an improvement in lipid profile and IR. These findings support the idea that RBEE could be considered as an exemplary candidate to be used as functional food in the treatment of the vascular complications associated with obesity.

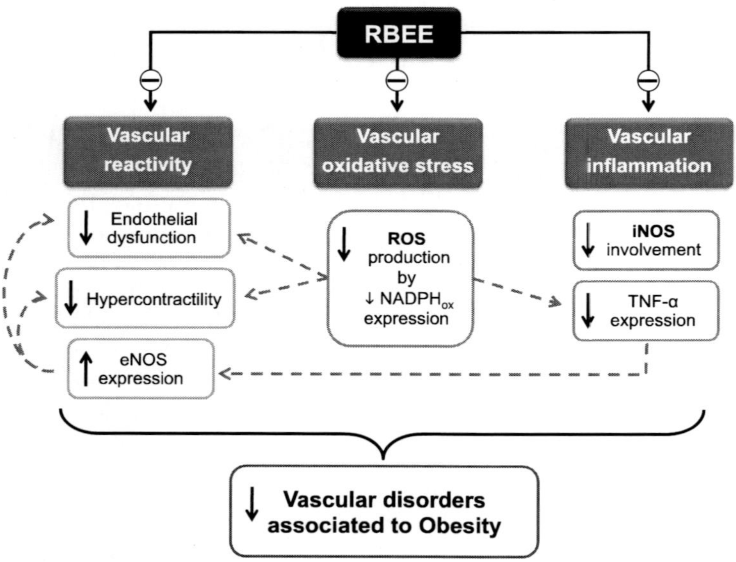

Figure 4. Schematic representation of mechanisms involved in the beneficial effects of RBEE in obesity-related vascular impairment. RBEE treatment attenuates vascular ROS production. This effect is related to a restoration of vascular reactivity by reducing endothelial dysfunction and hypercontractility as well as up-regulating eNOS expression. Also, RBEE attenuates vascular inflammation by reducing iNOS and TNF-α involvement, thus contributing to the improvement of vascular disorders associated with obesity. NADPHox, nicotinamide adenine dinucleotide phosphate-oxidase.

2.5.3. RBEE Restores Microvascular Dysfunction

In obesity, microvascular dysfunction may affect both peripheral vascular resistance and insulin-mediated glucose disposal, thereby contributing to hypertension and IR, respectively [114]. In our study, there was an evidently impaired NO contribution to vasodilatation in small mesenteric arteries (SMA) in obese rats [22]. This fact could be related to the up-regulation that RBEE administration induced in eNOS vascular expression. Our results agree with previous research where, despite the lack of changes in vasodilatation to ACh between lean and obese Zucker rats, there was a reduced inhibitory effect in the dilatation of small mesenteric arteries (SMA) in obese rats after simultaneous inhibition of COX and endothelial-derived hyperpolarizing factor responses compared to lean rats [115].

Experimental studies suggest that the contribution of endothelial derived hyperpolarizing factor (EDHF) increases as the vessel size decreases, with predominant activity in resistance arteries and a compensatory up-regulation of EDHF in states characterized by reduced NO availability [116]. For this reason, the restored EDHF contribution observed in small mesenteric arteries (SMA) in obese animals fed RBEE-supplemented diets could be an alternative resource for counteracting the loss of NO availability in these animals. EDHF has been shown to be particularly important in microcirculation, where systemic vascular resistance is regulated [116, 117]. EDHF impairment has been related to the metabolic disorders characteristic in obese Zucker rats, especially glucose and insulin alterations [118, 119]. These results could be associated to the beneficial effects of RBEE on IR demonstrated in obese Zucker rats [18]. Also, the effect of RBEE-diets on NO and EDHF contribution could contribute to the improvement in systolic blood pressure levels, through an enhanced peripheral vascular function [119, 120], observed in obese Zucker rats fed RBEE-diets.

Many lines of evidences suggest that increased vascular oxidative stress plays an important role in endothelial dysfunction and, in turn, in the impairment of NO/EDHF-mediated relaxation and the development of cardiovascular disease [115, 121]. Vascular depolarization leads to O_2 production and a reduction in NO bioavailability [122]. An RBEE-enriched diet induced a significant attenuation of O_2 production in SMA in obese Zucker rats that could be closely linked to the significant restoration of Ca^{2+}-activated K^+ (KCa) channels, as well as EDHF contribution induced by this dietary supplement.

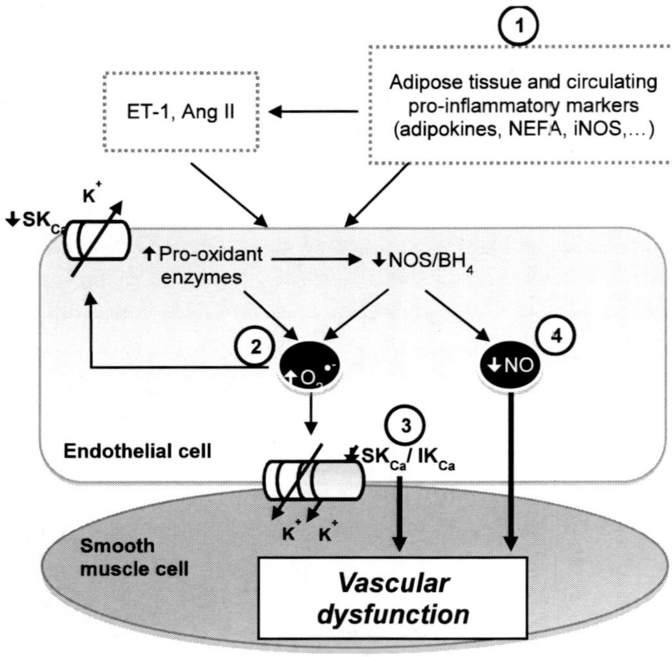

Figure 5. Representation of the mechanisms involved in the effects of RBEE in the dysfunction of small resistance arteries in obesity. Administration of RBEE attenuates inflammatory markers from adipose tissue (1) with the subsequent attenuation in vascular superoxide anion (2), increased levels of NO (3) and the restoration of calcium-activated potassium channels activation to maintain the EDH-response in the vasodilatation (4).

Abdominal obesity is closely associated with microvascular dysfunction, through indirect mechanisms, such as IR and directly due to the production of adipokines and pro-inflammatory cytokines by the perivascular adipose tissue, which in turns induce oxidative stress [114, 123, 124]. Administering an RBEE-supplemented diet restored levels of these inflammatory indicators in both adipose tissue and aorta in obese Zucker rats [21]. Similarly RBEE-diet attenuated iNOS expression in resistance arteries in obese rats, suggesting the anti-inflammatory potential of this treatment in obesity. The beneficial effect of RBEE against inflammation in adipose tissue might be related to the improved profile of inflammatory indicators in microvessels.

To summarize, RBEE-supplementation was able to restore microvascular function in obese Zucker rats by increasing the EDHF contribution throughout upregulation of endothelial small-conductance and intermediate-conductance, calcium-activated potassium channels (endothelial SKCa and IKCa channels) and a partial increase of NO bioavailability from eNOS, both mechanisms acting as a compensatory response against metabolic and vascular disorders in obesity. This positive effect was associated with a significant reduction of superoxide production and iNOS expression in the vascular wall. The beneficial effects of RBEE on inflammatory markers from visceral adipose tissue could play a critical role on these microvascular responses (Figure 5).

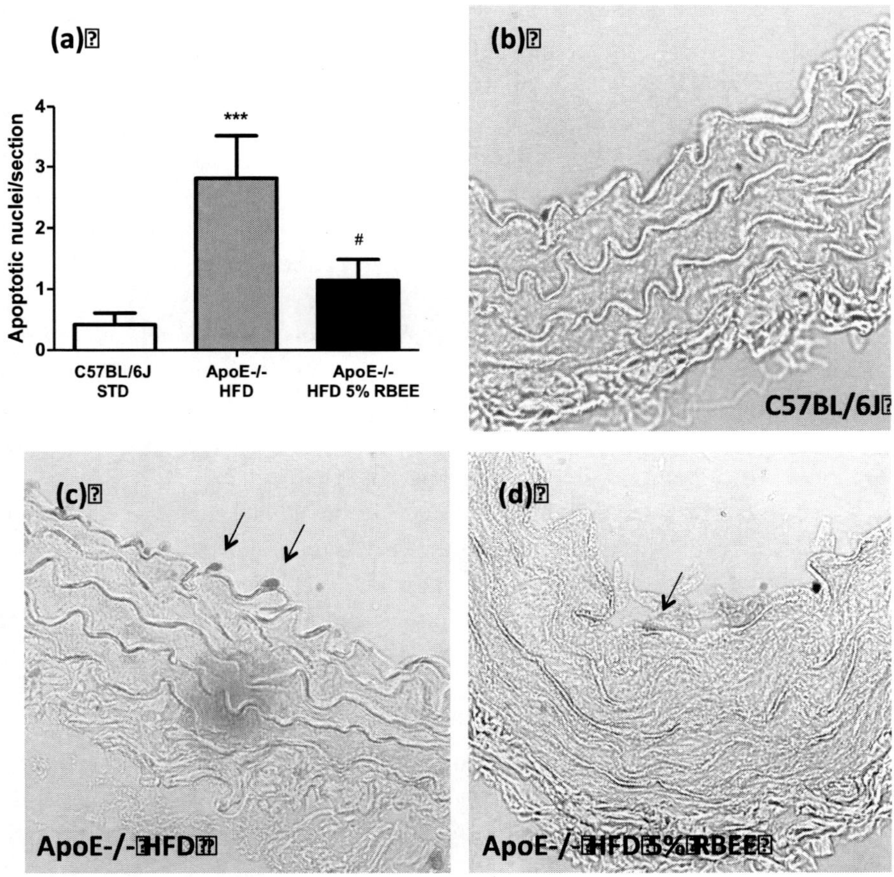

Figure 6. Histological determination of endothelial apoptosis. Five-micrometer paraffin embedded sections of the thoracic aorta were used for in situ determination of endothelial apoptosis. Arrows show positive apoptotic nuclei. (a) Quantification of apoptotic nuclei per section. Representative sections of (b) C57BL/6J, (c) ApoE−/− HFD and d ApoE−/− HFD 5% RBEE groups. RBEE reduced the number of apoptotic nuclei per ring ($^{\#}P < 0.05$, ApoE−/− HFD 5% RBEE *vs* ApoE−/− HFD; $^{***}P < 0.001$ ApoE−/− HFD *vs* C57BL/6J). Values are mean ± SEM of 8 (C57BL/6J)–9 (ApoE−/−) animals.

These results are in agreement with our observations showing the ability of RBEE- supplementation to ameliorate metabolic syndrome-related disorders such as dyslipidemia, insulin resistance, hypertension and vascular impairment of large conductance arteries [18, 21].

RBEE-supplementation also has beneficial effects on endothelial impairment of ApoE-/- mice [24]. We found that RBEE-supplementation has beneficial effects on the endothelium-dependent relaxation of ApoE-/-mice, revealing NO release by eNOS and oxidative stress amelioration as the main mechanisms. EDHF was found to be the main contributor to ACh-induced response in wild type C57BL/6J mice while NO was for ApoE-/- mice. In addition, the RBEE treatment was able to ameliorate remodeling in ApoE-/- mice, presenting itself as an interesting nutraceutical ingredient in the control of atherosclerotic-related disorders.

2.5.4. RBEE Protects against Cellular Senescence and Apoptosis in the Vascular Wall

RBEE-supplemented diets also protected against cellular senescence and apoptosis in the vascular wall and it potently prevents the development of atherosclerotic plaques in ApoE-/- mice (Figure 6) [23]. These effects were associated with improved serum lipid profiles and reduced telomere shortening in the vessel wall and in spleen-derived mononuclear cells.

Because RBEE is rich in antioxidant components such as γ-oryzanol, ferulic acid, tocols and sulfur amino acids (cysteine and methionine), which are precursors of the antioxidants taurine and glutathione [14, 16]. RBEE has the capacity to prevent lipid peroxidation and protein oxidation *in vitro* and *ex vivo* through scavenging hydroxyl and peroxyl radicals [29, 15]. Therefore, it can decrease oxidative stress which accelerates erosion and loss of telomeric DNA [125].

In atherosclerotic lesions, macrophage accumulation is correlated with plaque development by an accumulation of cholesterol and fatty acids. Therefore, macrophage apoptosis may have a positive effect in terms of the stability and progression of atherosclerotic lesions [126, 127]. The increased apoptosis of spleen mononuclear cell (MNC) induced by an RBEE-supplemented diet may disrupt macrophage development, leading to lower infiltration and plaque growth.

Interestingly, RBEE had a dual and opposite effect on MNC and aorta. RBEE provided remarkable telomere protection in MNC and aorta, but enhanced apoptosis in MNC, while it simultaneously reduced apoptosis in the aorta. Such differences could be attributed to one of the components of RBEE, namely tocopherols, which have been found to display pro-apoptotic and anti-proliferative effects upon cells with a high turnover such as in carcinogenic tissues while having low or no effects in non-malignant cells [128]. This dual effect may be a novel mechanism for the observed reduction in macrophage infiltration and plaque development.

The multi-factorial properties of RBEE-diet in the prevention of vascular alterations and the mechanisms mediating these actions, involve potential advantages over pharmacological strategies to treat cardio-vascular complications.

CONCLUSION

In conclusion, we describe in this chapter how enzymatic technology enables us to obtain a stable, water-soluble extract that preserves the main bioactive components in the original RB. We also describe the beneficial properties of RBEE in preventing and treating dysfunctions associated with oxidative stress and inflammatory response. These alterations are present in chronic diseases that are a major concern in modern societies.

REFERENCES

[1] National Research Council Committee on Diet and Health. *Diet and health: implications for reducing chronic disease risk*. 1989. National Academy of Sciences Press: Washington, DC., USA.

[2] Goufo P, Trindade H. Rice antioxidants: phenolic acids, flavonoids, anthocyanins, proanthocyanidins, tocopherols, tocotrienols, γ-oryzanol, and phytic acid. *Food Sci Nutr* 2, 75–104, 2014.

[3] Jariwalla RJ. Rice-bran products: phytonutrients with potential applications in preventive and clinical medicine. *Drugs Exp Clin Res* 27, 17–26, 2001.

[4] Qureshi AA, Sami SA, Khan FA. Effects of stabilized rice bran, its soluble and fiber fractions on blood glucose levels and serum lipid parameters in humans with diabetes mellitus types I and II. *J Nutr Biochem* 13, 175–187, 2002.

[5] Xu Z, Hua N, Godber JS. Antioxidant activity of tocopherols, tocotrienols, and γ-oryzanol components from rice bran against cholesterol oxidation accelerated by 2, 2-azobis (2-methyl propionamidine) dihydrochloride. *J Agr Food Chem* 49, 2077–2081, 2001.

[6] Islam MS1, Nagasaka R, Ohara K, Hosoya T, Ozaki H, Ushio H, Hori M. Biological abilities of rice bran-derived antioxidant phytochemicals for medical therapy. *Curr Top Med Chem* 11(14), 1847-53, 2011.

[7] Viriyaroj A, Ngawhirunpat T, Sukma M, Akkaramongkolporn P, Ruktanonchai U, Opanasopit P. Physicochemical properties and antioxidant activity of gamma-oryzanol-loaded liposome formulations for topical use. *Pharm Dev Technol*, 14, 665-671, 2009.

[8] Kennedy G, Burlingame B. Analysis of food composition data on rice from a plant genetic resources perspective. *Food Chem* 80, 589–596, 2003.

[9] Tsuji H, Kimoto M, Natori Y. Allergens in major crops. *Nutr Res* 21, 925–934, 2001.

[10] Morita T, Oh-Hashi A, Takei K, Ikai K, Kasaoka M, Kiriyama S. Cholesterol-lowering effects of soybean, potato and rice proteins depend on their low methionine contents in rats fed a cholesterol-free purified diet. *J Nutr* 127, 470–477, 1997.

[11] Sharif MK, Butt MS, Anjum FM, Afizkhan SH. Rice bran: A novel functional ingredient. *Crit Rev Food Sci* 54, 807–816, 2014.

[12] Nam SH, Choi SP, Kang MY, Kozukue N, Friedman M. Antioxidative, antimutagenic, and anticarcinogenic activities of rice bran extracts in chemical and cell assays. *J Agric Food Chem* 53, 816-822, 2005.

[13] Hagl S, Berressem D, Bruns B, Sus N, Frank J, Eckert GP. Beneficial effects of ethanolic and hexanic rice bran extract on mitochondrial function in PC12 cells and the search for bioactive components. *Molecules* 20(9), 16524-16539, 2015.

[14] Parrado J, Miramontes E, Jover M, Gutiérrez JF, Collantes de Terán L, Bautista J. Preparation of a rice bran enzymatic extract with potential use as functional food. *Food Chem* 98(4), 742-748, 2006.

[15] Santa María C, Revilla E, Miramontes E, Bautista J, García-Martínez A, Romero E, Carballo M, Parrado J. Protection against free radicals (UVB irradiation) of a water-soluble enzymatic extract from rice bran. Study using human keratinocyte monolayer and reconstructed human epidermis. *Food Chem Toxicol* 48, 83–88, 2010.

[16] Revilla E, Santa María C, Miramontes E, Bautista J, García-Martínez A, Cremades O, Cert R, Parrado P. Nutraceutical composition, antioxidant activity and hypocholesterolemic effect of a water-soluble enzymatic extract from rice bran. *Food Res Inter* 42, 387–393, 2009.

[17] Revilla E, Santa María C, Miramontes E, Candiracci M, Rodríguez-Morgado B, Carballo M, Bautista J, Castaño A, Parrado J. Antiproliferative and immunoactivatory ability of an enzymatic extract from rice bran. *Food Chem* 136, 526–531, 2013.

[18] Justo ML, Rodríguez–Rodríguez R, Claro CM, Álvarez de Sotomayor M, Parrado P, Herrera MD. Water-soluble rice bran enzymatic extract attenuates dyslipidemia, hypertension and insulin resistance in obese Zucker rats. *Eur J Nutr* 52, 789–797, 2013.

[19] Justo ML, Claro C, Zeyda M, Stulnig TM, Herrera MD, Rodriguez-Rodriguez R. Rice bran prevents high fat diet induced inflammation and macrophage content in adipose tissue. *Eur J Nutr* 55, 2011-2019, 2016.

[20] Candiracci M, Justo ML, Castaño A, Rodriguez-Rodriguez R, Herrera MD. Rice bran enzymatic extract–supplemented diets modulate adipose tissue inflammation markers in Zucker rats. *Nutrition* 30, 466–472, 2014.

[21] Justo ML, Candiracci M, Dantas AP, de Sotomayor M, Parrado J, Vila E, Herrera MD, Rodriguez-Rodriguez R. Rice bran enzymatic extract restores endothelial function and vascular contractility in obese rats by reducing vascular inflammation and oxidative stress. *J Nutr Biochem* 24, 1453–1461, 2013.

[22] Justo ML, Claro C, Vila E, Herrera MD, Rodriguez-Rodriguez R. Microvascular disorders in obese Zucker rats are restored by a rice bran diet. *Nutr Metabol Cardiov Dis* 24, 524-531, 2014.

[23] Pérez-Ternero C, Herrera MD, Laufs U, Alvarez de Sotomayor M, Werner CL. Food supplementation with rice bran enzymatic extract prevents vascularapoptosis and atherogenesis in ApoE-/- mice. *Eur J Nutr* http://dx.doi.org/10.1007/s00394-015-1074-z [Epub ahead of print].

[24] Pérez-Ternero C, Rodriguez-Rodríguez R, Herrera MD, Alvarez de Sotomayor M. Diet supplementation with rice bran enzymatic extract restoresendothelial impairment and wall remodelling of ApoE/mice microvessels. *Atherosclerosis* 250, 15-22, 2016.

[25] Adler-Nissen J. ISSPH-The production and properties of an enzymic food protein hydrolysate. pp. 263–313. In: *Enzymic hydrolysis of food proteins*. 1986. London, New York: Elsevier Applied Science Publisher.

[26] Parrado J, Bautista J, Machado A. Production of soluble enzymatic protein hydrolizate from industrially deffated undehulled sunflower meal. *J Agr Food Chem* 39, 447–450, 1991.

[27] Santa María C, Revilla E, García-Morgado B, Castaño A, Carbonero P, Gordillo B, Certz R, Parrado J. Effect of rice parboiling on the functional properties of an enzymatic extract from rice bran. *J Cer Sci* 72, 54-59, 2016.

[28] Halliwell B. Free radicals and antioxidants: updating a personal view. *Nutr Rev* 70, 257-265, 2012.

[29] Parrado J, Miramontes E, Jover M, Márquez JC, Mejias M, Collantes de Terán L, Absi E, Bautista J. Prevention of brain protein and lipid oxidation elicited by a water soluble oryzanol enzymatic extract derived from rice bran. *Eur J Nutr* 42, 307–314, 2003.

[30] Srinivasan M, Sudheer AR, Menon VP. Ferulic Acid: Therapeutic potential through its antioxidant property. *J Clin Biochem Nutr* 40, 92–100, 2007.

[31] Moreno-Gimenez JC, Bueno J, Navas J, Camacho F. Treatment of skin ulcer using oil of mosqueta rose. *Med Cutan Ibero Lat Am* 18, 63–66, 1990.

[32] Cao X, Ito Y. Supercritical fluid extraction of grape seed oil and subsequent separation of free fatty acids by high-speed counter-current chromatography. *J Chromatogr A* 1021, 117–124, 2003.

[33] Bonina F, Puglia C, Avogadro M, Baranelli E, Cravotto G. The topical protective effect of soybean-germ oil against UVB-Induced cutaneous erythema: an *in vivo* evaluation. *Arch Pharm Chem Life Sci* 338, 598–601, 2005.

[34] Lin FH, Lin JY, Gupta RD, Tournas JA, Burch JA, Selim MA. Ferulic acid stabilizes a solution of vitamins C and E and doubles its photoprotection of skin. *J Invest Dermatol* 125, 826–832, 2005.

[35] Tournas JA, Lin FH, Burch JA, Selim MA, Monteiro-Riviere NA, Zielinski JE. Ubiquinone, idebenone, and kinetin provide ineffective photoprotection to skin when compared to a topical antioxidant combination of vitamins C and E with ferulic acid. *J Invest Dermatol* 126, 1185–1187, 2006.

[36] Murray JC, Burch JA, Streilein RD, Iannacchione MA, Hall RP, Pinnell SR. A topical antioxidant solution containing vitamins C and E stabilized by ferulic acid provides protection for human skin against damage caused by ultraviolet irradiation. *J Am Acad Dermatol* 59, 418–425, 2008.

[37] Anand P, Kunnumakara AB, Sundaram C, Harikumar KB, Tharakan ST, Lai OS. Cancer is a preventable disease that requires major lifestyle changes. *Pharmac Res* 25, 2097–2116, 2008.

[38] Willett WC. Balancing life-style and genomics research for disease prevention. *Science* 296, 695–698, 2002.

[39] Minami M, Matsumoto S, Horiuchi H. Cardiovascular side-effects of modern cancer therapy. *Circulation J* 74, 1779–1786, 2010.

[40] Finkel T. Intracellular redox regulation by the family of small GTPases. *Antiox Redox Signal* 8, 1857–1863, 2006.

[41] Manda G, Nechifor, MT, Neagu TM. Reactive oxygen species. Cancer and anti-cancer therapies. *Current Chem Biol* 3, 342–366, 2009.

[42] Yu W, Simmons-Menchaca M, Gapor A, Sanders BG, Kline K. Induction of apoptosis in human breast cancer cells by tocopherols and tocotrienols. *Nutr Cancer* 33, 26–32, 1999.

[43] Nagasaka R, Chotimarkorn C, Shafiqul I, Hori M, Ozaki H, Ushio H. Antiinflammatory effects of hydroxycinnamic acid derivatives. *Biochem Biophys Res Commun* 358, 615–619, 2007.

[44] Ghoneum M, Matsuura M. Augmentation of macrophage phagocytosis by modified arabinoxylan rice bran (MGN-3/biobran). *Int J Immunopathol Pharm* 17, 283–292, 2004.

[45] Bruce KD, Hanson MA. The developmental origins, mechanisms and implications of metabolic syndrome. *J Nutr* 140, 648–652, 2010.

[46] Eckel RH, Grundy SM, Zimmet PZ. The metabolic syndrome. *Lancet* 365, 1415–1428, 2005.

[47] Alberti KG, Eckel RH, Grundy SM, Zimmet PZ, Cleeman JI, Donato KA, Fruchart JC, James WP, Loria CM, Smith SC Jr; International Diabetes Federation Task Force on Epidemiology and Prevention; Hational Heart, Lung, and Blood Institute; American Heart Association; World Heart Federation; International Atherosclerosis Society; International Association for the Study of Obesity. Harmonizing the metabolic syndrome: a joint interim statement of the International Diabetes Federation Task Force on Epidemiology and Prevention; National Heart, Lung, and Blood Institute; American Heart Association; World Heart Federation; International Atherosclerosis Society; and International Association for the Study of Obesity. *Circulation* 120(16), 1640–1645, 2009.

[48] Wang O, Liu J, Cheng Q, Guo X, Wang Y, Zhao L, Zhou F, Ji B. Effects of ferulic acid and γ-oryzanol on high-fat and high-fructose diet-induced metabolic syndrome in rats. *PLoS ONE* 2015;10(2)e0118135. doi:10.1371/journal.pone.0118135.

[49] Davi G, Santilli F, Patrono C. Nutraceuticals in diabetes and metabolic syndrome. *Cardiovasc Ther* 28, 216–226, 2010.

[50] Abete I, Goyenechea E, Zulet MA, Martínez JA. Obesity and metabolic syndrome: potential benefit from specific nutritional components. *Nutr Metab Cardiovasc Dis* 21(Suppl 2), B1–B15, 2011.

[51] Sharma RD, Rukmini C. Hypocholesterolemic activity of unsaponifiable fraction of rice bran oil. *Indian J Med Res* 85, 278- 281, 1987.

[52] Nicolosi RJ, Ausman LM, Hegsted DM. Rice bran oil lowers serum total and low density lipoprotein cholesterol and apo B levels in nonhuman primates. *Atherosclerosis* 88, 133-142, 1991.

[53] Yoshino G, Kazumi T, Amano M, Tateiwa M, Yamasaki T, Takashima S, Iwai, M, Hatanaka, H, Baba, S. Effects of gamma-oryzanol on hyperlipidemic subjects. *Cur Ther Res Clin Exp (USA)* 45, 543- 552, 1989.

[54] Theriault A, Chao J, Wang Q, Gapor A, Adeli K. Tocotrienol: a review of its therapeutic potential. *Clin Biochem* 32, 309- 319, 1999.

[55] Parker RA, Pearce BC, Clark RW, Gordon DA, Wright JJK. Tocotrienols regulate cholesterol production in mammalian cells by post-transcriptional suppression of 3-hydroxy-3-methyllutaryl coenzyme A reductase. *J Biol Chem* 268, 11230-11238, 1993.

[56] Qureshi AA, Bradlow BA, Brace L, Manganello J, Peterson DM, Pearce BC, Wright JJ, Gapor A, Elson CE. Response of hypercholesterolemic subjects to administration of tocotrienols. *Lipids* 30(12), 1171-1177, 1995.

[57] Mensink RP, Van Houwelingen AC, Kromhout D, Honstra G. A vitamin-E concentrate rich in tocotrienols had no effect on serum, lipoproteins, or platelet function in men with mildly elevated serum lipid concentrations. *Am J Clin Nutr* 69, 213-219, 1999.

[58] Wahlqvist ML, Krivokuca-Bogetic Z, Lo CH, Hage B, Smith R, Lukito, W. Differential serum response to tocopherols and tocotrienols during vitamin E supplementation in hypercholesterolemic individuals without change in coronary risk factors. *Nutr Res* 12, 181S-201S, 1992.

[59] Rogers EJ, Rice SM, Nicolosi RJ, Carpenter DR, McClelland CA, Romanczyk LJ. Identification and quantitation of γ-oryzanol components and simultaneous assessment of tocols in rice bran oil. *J Am Oil Chem Soc* 70, 301-307, 1993.

[60] Puchau B, Zulet MA, de Echávarri AG, Hermsdorff HH, Martínez JA. Dietary total antioxidant capacity is negatively associated with some metabolic syndrome features in healthy young adults. *Nutrition* 26, 534–541, 2010.

[61] Ha T-Y, Han S, Kim S-R, Kim I-H, Lee H-Y, Kim H-K. Bioactive components in rice bran oil improve lipid profiles in rats fed a high-cholesterol diet. *Nutr Res* 25, 597–606, 2005.

[62] Cicero AF, Gaddi A. Rice bran oil and gamma-oryzanol in the treatment of hyperlipoproteinaemias and other conditions. *Phytother Res* 15, 277–289, 2001.

[63] Ausman LM, Rong N, Nicolosi RJ. Hypocholesterolemic effect of physically refined rice bran oil: studies of colesterol metabolism and early atherosclerosis in hypercholesterolemic hamsters. *J Nutr Biochem* 16, 521–529, 2005.

[64] Berger A, Rein D, Schäfer A, Monnard I, Gremaud G, Lambelet P, Bertoli C. Similar cholesterol-lowering properties of rice bran oil, with varied gamma-oryzanol, in mildly hypercholesterolemic men. *Eur J Nutr* 44, 163–173, 2005.

[65] Wilson TA, Nicolosi RJ, Woolfrey B, Kritchevsky D. Rice bran oil and oryzanol reduce plasma lipid and lipoprotein colesterol concentrations and aortic cholesterol ester accumulation to a greater extent than ferulic acid in hypercholesterolemic hamsters. *J Nutr Biochem* 18, 105–112, 2007.

[66] Wang Y-K, Li Y, Sun A-M, Wang F-J, Yu G-P. Hypolipidemic and antioxidative effects of aqueous enzymatic extract from rice bran in rats fed a high-fat and -cholesterol diet. *Nutrients* 6, 3696-3710, 2014.

[67] Wilson TA, Idreis HM, Taylor CM, Nicolosi RJ. Whole fat rice bran reduces the development of early aortic atherosclerosis in hypercholesterolemic hamsters compared with wheat bran. *Nutrition Research* 22, 1319–1332, 2002.

[68] Scoggan KA, Gruber H, Chen Q, Plouffe LJ, Lefebvre JM, Wang B, Bertinato J, L'Abbé MR, Hayward S, Ratnayake WM. Increased incorporation of dietary plant sterols and cholesterol correlates with decreased expression of hepatic and intestinal ABCG5 and ABCG8 in diabetic BB rats. *J Nutr Biochem* 20(3), 177-186, 2009.

[69] Pérez-Ternero C, Bermúdez Pulgarín B, Alvarez de Sotomayor M, Herrera MD. Atherosclerosis-related inflammation and oxidative stress are improved by rice bran enzymatic extract. *Journal of Functional Foods* 26, 610–621, 2016.

[70] Kiribuchi M, Miura K, Tokuda S, Kaneda T. Hypocholesterolemic effect of triterpene alcohols with soy sterol on plasma cholesterol in rats. *J Nutr Science Vitamin* 29, 35–43, 1983.

[71] Minhajuddin M, Beg ZH, Iqbal J. Hypolipidemic and antioxidant properties of tocotrienol rich fraction isolated from rice bran oil in experimentally induced hyperlipidemic rats. *Food Chem Toxicol* 43, 747–753, 2005.

[72] Qureshi AA, Sami SA, Salser WA, Khan FA. Dose dependent suppression of serum cholesterol by tocotrienol-rich fraction (TRF25) of rice bran in hypercholesterolemic humans. *Atherosclerosis* 161, 199–207, 2002.

[73] Fabian C, Ju YH. A review on rice bran protein: its properties and extraction methods. *Crit Rev Food Sci Nutr* 51, 816–827, 2011.

[74] Ni W, Tsuda Y, Takashima S, Sato H, Sato M, Imaizumi K. Anti-atherogenic effect of soya and rice-protein isolate, compared with casein, in apolipoprotein E-deficient mice. *Br J Nutr* 90, 13–20, 2003.

[75] Tousoulis D, Böger RH, Antoniades C, Siasos G, Stefanadis E, Stefanadis C. Mechanisms of disease: L-arginine in coronary atherosclerosis – A clinical perspective. *Nat Clin Pract Card* 4, 274–283, 2007.

[76] Padmalayam I, Suto M. Role of adiponectin in the metabolic syndrome: current perspectives on its modulation as a treatment strategy. *Curr Pharm Des* 19, 5755–5763, 2013.

[77] Grundy SM. Metabolic syndrome update. *Trends Cardiovasc Med* 26, 364-373, 2016.

[78] Taskinen MR, Boren J. New insights into the pathophysiology of dyslipidemia in type 2 diabetes. *Atherosclerosis* 239, 483–495, 2015.

[79] Chen CW, Cheng HH. A rice bran oil diet increases LDL receptor and HMG-CoA reductase mRNA expressions and insulin sensitivity in rats with streptozotocin/nicotinamideinduced type 2 diabetes. *J Nutr* 136, 1472–1476, 2006.

[80] Chou TW, Ma CY, Cheng HH, Chen YY, Lai MH. A rice bran oil diet improves lipid abnormalities and suppress hyperinsulinemic responses in rats with streptozotocin/nicotinamide induced type 2 diabetes. *J Clin Biochem Nutr* 45, 29–36, 2009.

[81] Siddiqui S, Rashid KM, Siddiqui WA. Comparative hypoglycemic and nephroprotective effects of tocotrienol rich fraction (TRF) from palm oil and rice bran oil against hyperglycemia induced nephropathy in type 1 diabetic rats. *Chem Biol Interact* 188(3), 651–658, 2010.

[82] Ruan H, Dong LQ. Adiponectin signaling and function in insulin target tissues. *J Mol Cell Biol* 8, 101–109, 2016.

[83] Ouchi N, Kihara S, Funahashi T, Matsuzawa Y, Walsh K. Obesity, adiponectin and vascular inflammatory disease. *Curr Opin Lipidol* 14, 561–566, 2003.

[84] Tilg H, Moschen, AR. Adipocytokines: Mediators linking adipose tissue, inflammation and immunity. *Nat Rev Immunol* 6, 772–783, 2006.

[85] Karalis KP, Giannogonas P, Kodela E, Koutmani Y, Zoumakis M, Thalia T. Mechanisms of obesity and related pathology: linking immune responses to metabolic stress. *FEBS J* 276, 5747-5754, 2009.

[86] Wang L, Gao S, Jiang W, Cheng L, Xu M, Bohlin L, Rosendahl M, Wenlin HW. Antioxidative dietary compounds modulate gene expression associated with apoptosis, DNA repair, inhibition of cell proliferation and migration. *Int J Mol Sci* 15, 16226-16245, 2014.

[87] Aleixandre de Artiñano A, Miguel Castro M. Experimental rat models to study the metabolic síndrome. *Br J Nutr* 102(9), 1246–1253, 2009.

[88] Kaileh M, Sen R. Role of NF-kappaB in the anti-inflammatory effects of tocotrienols. *J Am Coll Nutr* 29, S334-S339, 2010.

[89] Wu SJ, Liu PL, Ng LT. Tocotrienol-rich fraction of palm oil exhibits anti-inflammatory property by suppressing the expression of inflammatory mediators in human monocytic cells. *Mol Nutr Food Res* 52, 921-929, 2008.

[90] Matsunaga T, Shoji A, Gu N, Joo E, Li S, Adachi T, Yamazaki H, Yasuda K, Kondoh T, Tsuda K. γ-tocotrienol attenuates TNF-α-induced changes in secretion and gene expression of MCP-1, IL-6 and adiponectin in 3 T3-L1 adipocytes. *Mol Med Report* 5(4), 905–909, 2012.

[91] Bluher M. Adipose tissue dysfunction in obesity. *Exp Clin Endocrinol Diabetes* 117, 241–250, 2009.

[92] Yang J, Eliasson B, Smith U, Cushman SW, Sherman AS. The size of large adipose cells is a predictor of insulin resistance in first-degree relatives of type 2 diabetic patients. *Obesity (Silver Spring)* 20(5), 932–938, 2012.

[93] Olefsky J, Glass C. Macrophages, inflammation, and insulin resistance. *Annu Rev Physiol* 72, 219–246, 2010.

[94] Ohashi K, Parker JL, Ouchi N, Higuchi A, Vita JA, Gokce N, Pedersen AA, Kalthoff C, Tullin S, Sams A, Summer R, Walsh K. Adiponectin promotes macrophage polarization toward an anti-inflammatory phenotype. *J Biol Chem* 285(9), 6153–6160, 2010.

[95] Kumada M, Kihara S, Ouchi N, Kobayashi H, Okamoto Y, Ohashi K, Maeda K, Nagaretani H, Kishida K, Maeda N, Nagasawa A, Funahashi T, Matsuzawa Y. Adiponectin specifically increased tissue inhibitor of metalloproteinase-1 through interleukin-10 expression in human macrophages. *Circulation* 109(17), 2046–2049, 2004.

[96] Nagasaka R, Yamsaki T, Uchida A, Ohara K, Ushio H. γ-Oryzanol recovers mouse hypoadiponectinemia induced by animal fat ingestion. *Phytomedicine* 18, 669–671, 2011.

[97] Imam M, Ismail M, Ithnin H, Tubesha Z, Omar A. Effects of germinated brown rice and its bioactive compounds on the expression of the peroxisome proliferator-activated receptor gamma gene. *Nutrients* 5, 468–477, 2013.

[98] Prasad K. Natural products in regression and slowing of progression of atherosclerosis. *Curr Pharm Biotechnol* 11, 794-800, 2010.

[99] Friedman M. Rice bran, rice bran oils, and rice hulls: composition, food and industrial uses, and bioactivities in humans, animals, and cells. *J Agric Food Chem* 61, 10626-10641, 2013.

[100] Haslam DW, James WP. Obesity. *Lancet* 366, 1197–1209, 2005.

[101] Kadowaki T, Yamauchi T, Kubota N, Hara K, Ueki K, Tobe K. Adiponectin and adiponectin receptors in insulin resistance, diabetes, and the metabolic syndrome. *J Clin Invest* 116, 1784–1792, 2006.

[102] Suzuki A, Kagawa D, Fujii A, Ochiai R, Tokimitsu I, Saito I. Short- and long-term effects of ferulic acid on blood pressure in spontaneously hypertensive rats. *Am J Hypertens* 15, 351–357, 2002.

[103] Ardiansyah SH, Koseki T, Hashizume K, Komai M. The Driselase-treated fraction of rice bran is a more effective dietary factor to improve hypertension, glucose and lipid metabolism in stroke-prone spontaneously hypertensive rats compared to ferulic acid. *Br J Nutr* 97(1), 67–76, 2007.

[104] Ardiansyah, Ohsaki Y, Shirakawa H, Koseki T, Komai M. Novel effects of a single administration of ferulic acid on the regulation of blood pressure and the hepatic lipid metabolic profile in stroke-prone spontaneously hypertensive rats. *J Agric Food Chem* 56(8), 2825–2830, 2008.

[105] Tesauro M, Schinzari F, Iantorno M, Rizza S, Melina D, Lauro D, Cardillo C. Ghrelin improves endothelial function in patients with metabolic syndrome. *Circulation* 112(19), 2986–2992, 2005.

[106] Frisbee JC. Impaired skeletal muscle perfusion in obese Zucker rats. *Am J Physiol Regul Integr Comp Physiol* 285(5), R1124–R1134, 2003.

[107] Janiak P, Lainee P, Grataloup Y, Luyt CE, Bidouard JP, Michel JB, O'Connor SE, Herbert JM. Serotonin receptor blockade improves distal perfusion after lower limb ischaemia in the fatty Zucker rat. *Cardiovasc Res* 56(2), 293–302, 2002.

[108] Wu SQ, Hopfner RL, McNeill JR, Wilson TW, Gopalakrishnan V. Altered paracrine effect of endothelin in blood vessels of the hyperinsulinemic, insulin resistant obese Zucker rat. *Cardiovasc Res* 45, 994–1000, 2000.

[109] Stepp DW, Frisbee JC. Augmented adrenergic vasoconstriction in hypertensive diabetic obese Zucker rats. *Am J Physiol Heart Circ Physiol* 282(3), H816–H820, 2002.

[110] Noronha BT, Li JM, Wheatcroft SB, Shah AM, Kearney MT. Inducible nitric oxide synthase has divergent effects on vascular and metabolic function in obesity. *Diabetes* 54, 1082–1089, 2005.

[111] Frisbee JC, Stepp DW. Impaired NO-dependent dilation of skeletal muscle arterioles in hypertensive diabetic obese Zucker rats. *Am J Physiol Heart Circ Physiol* 281, H1304–H1311, 2001.

[112] Landmesser U, Cai H, Dikalov S, McCann L, Hwang J, Jo H, Holland SM, Harrison DG. Role of p47(phox) in vascular oxidative stress and hypertension caused by angiotensin II. *Hypertension* 40(4), 511–515, 2002.

[113] Matsuno K, Yamada H, Iwata K, Jin D, Katsuyama M, Matsuki M, Takai S, Yamanishi K, Miyazaki M, Matsubara H, Yabe-Nishimura C. Nox1 is involved in angiotensin II-mediated hypertension: a study in Nox1-deficient mice. *Circulation* 112(17), 2677–2685, 2005.

[114] Hornstra JM, Serné EH, Eringa EC, Wijnker MC, de Boer MP, Yudkin JS, Smulders YM. Insulin's microvascular vasodilatory effects are inversely related to peripheral vascular resistance in overweight, but insulin-sensitive subjects. *Obesity (Silver Spring)* 21(12), 2557-2561, 2013.

[115] Agouni A, Lagrue-Lak-Hal AH, Mostefai HA, Tesse A, Mulder P, Rouet P, Desmoulin F, Heymes C, Martínez MC, Andriantsitohaina R. Red wine polyphenols prevent metabolic and cardiovascular alterations associated with obesity in Zucker fatty rats (Fa/Fa). *PLoS One* 4, e5557, 2009. doi: 10.1371/journal.pone.0005557.

[116] Ozkor MA, Quyyumi AA. Endothelium-derived hyperpolarizing factor and vascular function. *Cardiol Res Pract* 2011, 156146, 2011. doi: 10.4061/2011/156146.

[117] Grgic I, Kaistha BP, Hoyer J, Köhler R. Endothelial Ca^{+}-activated K^{+} channels in normal and impaired EDHF-dilator responses-relevance to cardiovascular pathologies and drug discovery. *Br J Pharmacol* 157, 509-526, 2009.

[118] Young EJ, Hill MA, Wiehler WB, Triggle CR, Reid JJ. Reduced EDHF responses and connexin activity in mesenteric arteries from the insulin-resistant obese Zucker rat. *Diabetologia* 51, 872-881, 2008.

[119] Burnham MP, Johnson IT, Weston AH. Impaired small-conductance Ca^{2+}-activated K^{+} channel-dependent EDHF responses in Type II diabetic ZDF rats. *Br J Pharmacol* 148, 434-441, 2006.

[120] Tesauro M, Cardillo C. Obesity, blood vessels and metabolic syndrome. *Acta Physiol (Oxf)* 203, 279-286, 2011.

[121] Cauwels A, Rogge E, Janssen B, Brouckaert P. Reactive oxygen species and small-conductance calcium-dependent potassium channels are key mediators of inflammation-induced hypotension and shock. *J Mol Med (Berl)* 88, 921-930, 2010.

[122] Gaete PS, Lillo MA, Ardiles NM, Pérez FR, Figueroa XF. Ca^{2+}-activated K^{+} channels of small and intermediate conductance control eNOS activation through NAD(P)H oxidase. *Free Radic Biol Med* 52, 860-870, 2012.

[123] Bagi Z, Feher A, Cassuto J. Microvascular responsiveness in obesity: implications for therapeutic intervention. *Br J Pharmacol* 165, 544-560, 2012.

[124] Virdis A, Neves MF, Duranti E, Bernini G, Taddei S. Microvascular endothelial dysfunction in obesity and hypertension. *Curr Pharm Des* 19, 2382-2389, 2013.

[125] von Zglinicki T. Oxidative stress shortens telomeres. *Trends Biochem Sci* 27, 339–344, 2002.

[126] Brown AL, Zhu X, Rong S, Shewale S, Seo J, Boudyguina E, Gebre AK, Alexander-Miller MA, Parks JS. Omega-3 fatty acids ameliorate atherosclerosis by favorably altering monocyte subsets and limiting monocyte recruitment to aortic lesions. *Arterioscler Thromb Vasc Biol* 32, 2122–2130, 2012.

[127] Dutta P, Courties G, Wei Y, Leuschner F, Gorbatov R, Robbins CS, Iwamoto Y, Thompson B, Carlson AL, Heidt T, Majmudar MD, Lasitschka F, Etzrodt M, Waterman P, Waring MT, Chicoine AT, van der Laan AM, Niessen HW, Piek JJ, Rubin BB, Butany J, Stone JR, Katus HA, Murphy SA, Morrow DA, Sabatine MS, Vinegoni C, Moskowitz MA, Pittet MJ, Libby P, Lin CP, Swirski FK, Weissleder R, Nahrendorf M. Myocardial infarction accelerates atherosclerosis. *Nature* 487(7407), 325–329, 2012.

[128] Henderson AJ, Ollila CA, Kumar A, Borresen EC, Raina K, Agarwal R, Ryan EP. Chemopreventive properties of dietary rice bran: current status and future prospects. *Adv Nutr* 3(5), 643–653, 2012.

In: Nutraceuticals
Editor: Noboru Motohashi
ISBN: 978-1-53611-785-1

Chapter 4

PHYTO-MELATONIN: A NATURAL SUBSTANCE FROM PLANTS WITH INTERESTING NUTRACEUTICAL PROPERTIES

Marino B. Arnao* and Josefa Hernández-Ruiz
Department of Plant Biology, University of Murcia,
Murcia, Spain

ABSTRACT

The main objective of this chapter is to provide information on a substance that has revolutionized studies in various scientific fields and is expected to have a great impact on the study of natural substances with nutraceutical properties. Phyto-melatonin (plant melatonin) is chemically related to amino acids but with very diverse properties. The interest in phyto-melatonin is due to its outstanding action at cellular and physiological level, while its plant origin offers many opportunities because it is a natural compound. An overview on its origin, its action in plants in general and in particular plant species with high levels of phyto-melatonin, and its use as a nutraceutical, is present. The beneficial effects that it may have on human health are also analyzed. The differences between synthetic melatonin and phyto-melatonin, according to their

* Corresponding author Email: marino@um.es.

origin and purity, will be presented. Finally, a brief discussion on the current market for phyto-melatonin and its limits and possibilities is presented.

Keywords: Antioxidant, cancer, cereals, circadian rhythm, free radicals, fruits, medicinal plants, melatonin, neurological diseases, nuts, nutraceutical, phyto-melatonin, plant foodstuffs, seeds, dietary/food supplements, vegetables

ABBREVIATIONS

CMH	Chinese medicinal herbs
CSF	cerebrospinal fluid
DW	dry weight
EMS	eosinophilia-myalgia syndrome
EU	European Union
FDA	Food and Drug Administration
FW	fresh weight
GC-MS	gas chromatography mass spectrometry
LC-MS	liquid chromatography mass spectrometry
RNS	reactive nitrogen species
ROS	reactive oxygen species
SCN	suprachiasmatic nucleus
SFE	supercritical fluid extraction
UV	ultraviolet

1. INTRODUCTION

The term phyto-melatonin was first proposed in 2004 in the scientific journal *Carcinogenesis,* in an article about the treatment of liver cancer in rats [1]. In this article, the possible use of phyto-melatonin from edible plants to arrest and counteract the progress of tumor liver cells was studied. According to the authors, *"... phyto-melatonin could have a potentially significant impact as a new strategy in human cancer prevention."*

Structurally, phyto-melatonin, as well as melatonin, is the compound *N*-acetyl-5-methoxytryptamine (Figure 1), an indoleamine derivative of other well-known compounds such as serotonin (neurotransmitter) and tryptophan (amino acid). While melatonin is the term used to refer to the compound of animal origin or from chemical synthesis, phyto-melatonin is the term used to refer to melatonin of a plant origin.

But, let's begin at the beginning. Phyto-melatonin was discovered in 1995 in higher plants, simultaneously by two research groups [2, 3], thirty seven years after the discovery of melatonin in bovine pineal gland by Lerner in 1958 [4] and in humans in 1959 [5]. From 1958 to 1995, it was thought that melatonin was a molecule exclusive to animals (mammals, fish, amphibians, birds), with a hormonal character and neurological activity in some cases. The discovery of the presence of melatonin in plants completely revolutionized our scientific view of this substance. Until that time was thought to be a highly evolved molecule that could only be found in animal species, but in the 1980s melatonin was discovered in invertebrates such as annelids, mollusks, insects and crustaceans [6-8]. The ubiquitous presence of phyto-melatonin in many plants analyzed opened up the possibility of investigating its possible role in totally different tissues and organs such as nerve tissue, liver, retina and gastrointestinal tract and also in roots, seeds, fruits or leaves of a plant. All tissues and organs of animals and plants have melatonin in greater or lesser amounts. Successive studies have quantified the presence of phyto-melatonin in plants, and it is now fully accepted that melatonin is present in all kingdoms, from prokaryotes to eukaryotes, from animals to plants. However, there are gaps where the molecule has not been studied, such as in lichens, or where scant information is available, as in fungi, bacteria and non-vascular plants [9-11].

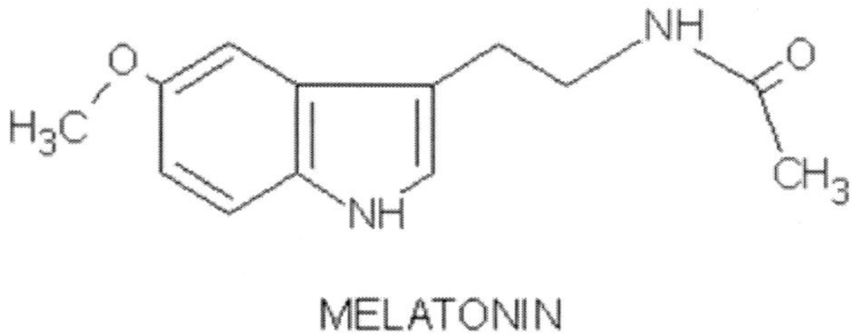

Figure 1. Molecular structure of melatonin (*N*-acetyl-5-methoxytryptamine).

2. PHYTO-MELATONIN IN PLANTS

Melatonin has been detected and quantified in roots, seedlings, shoots, leaves, flowers, fruits and seeds of a considerable variety of plant species, especially in edible plants.

Tables 1, 2, 3, 4, 5 and 6 summarize some of the data available to date for fruits, vegetables, cereals, beverages, seeds/nuts and medicinal plants, respectively, with a known high phyto-melatonin content. Among fruits (Table 1), goji berries, a very small berry with very interesting properties, show the highest phyto-melatonin content [12]. Any attempt at classification according to the phyto-melatonin content is very difficult, because the data are highly variable. However, taking the maximum levels observed in the quantification analysis for each species, the Rosaceae family, i.e., apple and cherries (sweet and tart), have a high content. Also, it is important to note that several varieties of *Vitis vinifera* have been seen to have a high phyto-melatonin content, a though there is a high degree of dispersion in the data. Most tropical fruits have low phyto-melatonin content. Among vegetables (Table 2), the Solanaceae family (tomatoes and pepper) has high phyto-melatonin content, as do *Brassica* species, although far below the above values. In cereals (Table 3), their contents range from 0.5 to 1.8 in the case of flours, a significant amount if we take into account our intake of these grains in the form of flour for baking. In the case of whole plants, data are more variable.

The phyto-melatonin content of coffee beans is of note (Table 4), surprisingly with a level that is about 6,000 times higher than that of cereal seeds. Roasted coffee beans have a higher phyto-melatonin content than green beans (~9 μg/g dry weight (DW)), and there is 60-78 ng of phyto-melatonin per mL of brewed coffee [13]. Red and white wines have lower phyto-melatonin content than beer and tea. In the case of seeds/nuts (Table 5), mustard seeds have high phyto-melatonin levels. Of note, too, are the levels in sunflower and alfalfa seeds. In aromatic/medicinal plants, thyme, liquorice root, sage and St. John's wort plants have very high levels (Table 6), higher than the content of coffee beans. Generally, Chinese medicinal herbs (CMH) have the highest phyto-melatonin content, but studies of medicinal plants of non-Chinese origin are scarce. Other medicinal plants such as feverfew (*Tanacetum parthenium*) also been seen to have high phyto-melatonin content.

Table 1. Content of phyto-melatonin in some fruits

Common Name/*Specie*	Phyto-melatonin content[1]	Ref.
Goji berry/*Lycium barbarum* L.	530	[14]
Apple/*Malus domestica* Borkh.	134	[15]
Sweet cherry/*Prunus avium* L.	120	[16]
Tart cherry/*Prunus cerasus* L.	14	[17]
Grape/*Vitis vinifera* L.	18	[18]
Strawberry/*Fragaria x ananassa* Duch.	12	[3]
Pomegranate/*Punica granatum* L.	5	[19]
Fig/*Ficus carica* L.	4	[20]
Orange/*Citrus x sinensis* L.	3	[21]
Mango/*Mangifera indica* L.	0.7	[22]
Banana/*Musa acuminate* Colla	0.6	[23]
Pineapple/*Ananas comosus* L.	0.3	[24]
Papaya/*Carica papaya* L.	0.2	[22]
Kiwifruit/*Actinidia deliciosa* Liang-Ferg	0.02	[3]

[1]Amounts expressed as nanograms (ng) of phyto-melatonin per gram of fresh edible tissue

Table 2. Content of phyto-melatonin in some vegetables

Common Name/Species	Phyto-melatonin content[1]	Ref.
Tomato/*Solanum lycopersicum* L.	114	[25]
Pepper (bell)/*Capsicum annuum* L.	42	[26]
Kohlrabi/*Brassica napus napobrassica*	7.8	[27]
Rutabaga/*Brassica oleracea acephala*	5.1	[27]
White radish/*Raphanus sativus* L.	0.6	[3]
Chinese cabbage/*Brassica rapa* L.	0.11	[3]
Cabbage/*Brassica oleracea capitata* L.	0.11	[3]
Welsh onion/*Allium fistulosum* L.	0.08	[3]
Carrot/*Daucus carota* Hoffm.	0.05	[3]
Onion/*Allium cepa* L.	0.03	[3]
Indian spinach/*Basella alba* L.	0.04	[3]
Cucumber/*Cucumis sativum* L.	0.02	[3]
Beetroot/*Beta vulgaris* L.	0.002	[2]

[1]Amounts expressed as nanograms (ng) per gram of fresh edible tissue

Table 3. Content of phyto-melatonin in some cereals

Common Name/Species	Phyto-melatonin content		Ref.
	Flour[1]	Whole plant[2]	
Oat/*Avena sativa* L.	1.8	90	[3, 28]
Sweet corn/*Zea mays* L.	1.3	--	[3]
Rice/*Oryza sativa* L.	1.0	0.3	[3]
Barley/*Hordeum vulgare* L.	0.5	50	[29]
Canarygrass/*Phalaris canariensis* L.	--	25	[28]
Wheat/*Triticum aestivum* L. (bread)	1.0 0.3	120	[29] [30]

[1]Amounts expressed as nanograms (ng) per gram of dry tissue
[2]Amounts expressed as nanograms (ng) per gram of fresh tissue

Table 4. Content of phyto-melatonin in some beverages

Common Name/Species	Phyto-melatonin content[1]	Ref.
Coffee beans/*Coffea sp.* Brewed coffee	6,500 60 (ml)	[13]
Mulberry leaves/*Morus sp.* Green tea Black tea	 46 40	[31]
Tea/*Camellia sinensis* L. Black Green	0.4 0.01	[1]
Cacao powder/*Theobroma cacao* L.	0.007	[30]
Grape (red)/*Vitis vinifera* L. Red wine White wine	18-0.01 0.31 (ml) 0.21 (ml)	[18] [32]
Beer/*Hordeum vulgare* L. Alcoholic beer Non-alcoholic beer	0.11 (ml) 0.05 (ml)	[30]
Orange juice/*Citrus x sinensis* L.	3.1 (ml)	[21]

[1]Amounts expressed as nanograms (ng) per gram of dry tissue (or per milliliter, mL)

Table 5. Content of phyto-melatonin in some seeds and nuts

Common Name/Species	Phyto-melatonin content[1]	Ref.
Jujube/*Ziziphus jujube* Lam.	256	[14]
White Mustard/*Brassica hirta* L.	189	[33]
Black Mustard/*Brassica nigra* L.	129	"
Fenugreek/*Trigonella foenum-graecum* L.	43	"
Almond/*Prunus amygdalus* Batsch.	39	"
Sunflower/*Helianthus annuus* L.	29	"
Fennel/*Foeniculum vulgare* Mill.	28	"
Alfalfa/*Medicago sativa* L.	16	"
Cardamom/*Elettaria cardamomum* L.	15	"
Flax/*Linum usitatissimum* L.	12	"
Cucumber/*Cucumis sativus* L.	11	[34]
Anise/*Pimpinella anisum* L.	7	[33]
Coriander/*Coriandrum sativum* L.	7	"
Lupin/*Lupinus albus* L.	3.8	[29]
Walnut/*Juglans regia* L.	3.5	[35]
Peanut/*Arachis hypogaea* L.	2.3	[1]
Milk thistle/*Sylibum marianum* L.	2	[33]
Olive oil/*Olea europaea* L.	0.1	[36]

[1]Amounts expressed as nanograms (ng) per gram of dry tissue

Table 6. Content of phyto-melatonin in some medicinal plants

Common Name/Species	Phyto-melatonin content[1]	Ref.
Thyme/*Thymus vulgaris* L.	38,000	[37]
Chinese liquorice/*Glycyrrhiza uralensis* Fisch.	34,000	[38]
Sage/*Salvia officinalis* L.	29,000	[37]
St. John's wort/*Hypericum perforatum* L.	23,000	[39]
Peppermint/*Mentha piperita*	19,500	[14]
Cat's claw herb/*Uncaria rhynchophylla* Miq.	2,460	[14]
Tokyo violet/*Viola philipica* Cav.	2,360	[14]
Feverfew/*Tanacetum parthenium* L.	1,700	[40]
Wolfberry/*Lycium barbarum* L.	530	[14]
Clove/*Syzygium aromaticum* L.	446	[14]
Korean mint/*Agastache rugosa* Kuntz.	300	[14]
Purslane/*Portulaca oleracea* L.	19	[41]
Laurel/*Laurus nobilis* L.	8	[20]

[1]Amounts expressed as nanograms (ng) per gram of dry tissue

2.1. Different Species, Different Plant Tissues, Different Cultivation Conditions, Different Phyto-Melatonin Contents

Since its discovery, one of the peculiarities observed in studies of phyto-melatonin has been the great disparity in the concentration of this substance. Thus, levels of phyto-melatonin from a few nanograms (ng) to quite considerable amounts, around micrograms (μg), per gram of plant tissue [42].

Generally, seeds, leaves, stems, seedlings and roots present the highest levels of phyto-melatonin and fruits the lowest. In general, aromatic and medicinal plants have significantly higher levels of phyto-melatonin than seed and fleshy fruits. However, there are only rough estimates because, depending on the varieties, growing conditions and other circumstances, the levels may vary. Nevertheless, the influence of harvest time and/or ripening stage is an important factor in determining the phyto-melatonin levels in some plant tissues but is decisive in the case of fruits. Generally, phyto-melatonin decreases as the fruit becomes more mature. Also, post-harvest conditions play a decisive role in phyto-melatonin levels, because of the influence of the hormone ethylene [29].

Environmental conditions (natural or artificial) are decisive factors regarding phyto-melatonin levels. Thus, light, temperature, soil humidity, air and soil toxics and ultraviolet (UV) radiation play a relevant role in the phyto-melatonin content of plants. Plants cultivated in field conditions tend to show a higher phyto-melatonin content than plants cultivated in growth chambers, where light, temperature and humidity are controlled automatically. For example, tomato plants cultivated in field conditions have up to 3-fold the phyto-melatonin level of those grown in culture chambers [43]. In general, phyto-melatonin levels increase in stress situations, protecting and strengthening the plants through an anti-stress response [11, 44]. For example, chemical toxic stressors such as heavy metals, saline solutions (NaCl) and hydrogen peroxide (H_2O_2) produce an up to 12-fold increase in phyto-melatonin levels in lupin and in barley plants [45, 46]. Also, a water deficit in soil provokes an increase in endogenous phyto-melatonin of between 2 and 4-fold the level observed in well-irrigated plants. This protective role of phyto-melatonin was observed, for example, in the resistance capacity of apple trees treated with exogenous melatonin to long-term drought stress [47].

2.2. Role of Phyto-Melatonin in Plants

Phyto-melatonin has been related with several aspects of plant physiology. The actions/activity of phyto-melatonin can be classified in two classes: those in which the indolamine acts as an antioxidant and those where it acts as a plant growth regulator (plant hormone) [44]. With respect to the first, the excellent properties of melatonin as antioxidant have been demonstrated in numerous studies, mainly in animals but also in plants. Phyto-melatonin can act as a direct antioxidant (Figure 2) through the stabilization of biological membranes, where it plays a relevant role in membrane fluidity and in counteracting lipid peroxidation. Also, phyto-melatonin acts by reducing oxidative stress through the redox network, modifying the expression of redox genes, among others, involved into the multiple anti-stress responses. Thus, the negative/deleterious effects on plants of abiotic stressors such as copper or zinc in soils, cold or high temperatures, herbicides or chemical toxicity, salinity, soil drought, light/dark and UV radiation and dark-induced leaf senescence can be reduced or minimized by the presence of phyto-melatonin [11, 48, 49]. Generally, these stress agents provoke an increase in endogenous phyto-melatonin levels, suggesting that it plays a significant physiological role in many stress situations, strengthening the cell redox-regulated network [46]. Also, its role as protector against biotic stressors such as pathogens is being studied. In general, phyto-melatonin provokes a protection response against several plant pathogens such as bacteria and fungi [50, 51].

With regard to the possible role of phyto-melatonin as plant hormone, the data indicate that phyto-melatonin acts in the same way as an auxin (plant hormone) in some situations (Figure 2). For example, in 2004, we demonstrated that it can promote the growth of etiolated lupin hypocotyls in the same way as auxin, a well-known plant hormone [52]. This growth promoting-activity was subsequently checked in other species, including several monocots, Brassicaceae and in rice plants [28, 44]. Another action of phyto-melatonin as a plant growth regulator was seen to be its capacity to induce changes in the rhizogenetic pattern. Thus, phyto-melatonin provokes the generation of adventitious and lateral roots in lupin plants, similarly to those induced by the hormone auxin [53]. This important effect also was later confirmed in cucumber, cherry rootstocks, rice seedlings, *Arabidopsis thaliana, Citrus sp.* and pomegranate. Phyto-melatonin also seems play some role in the modulation of organogenesis in culture explants and in flowering and fruit development [11, 54].

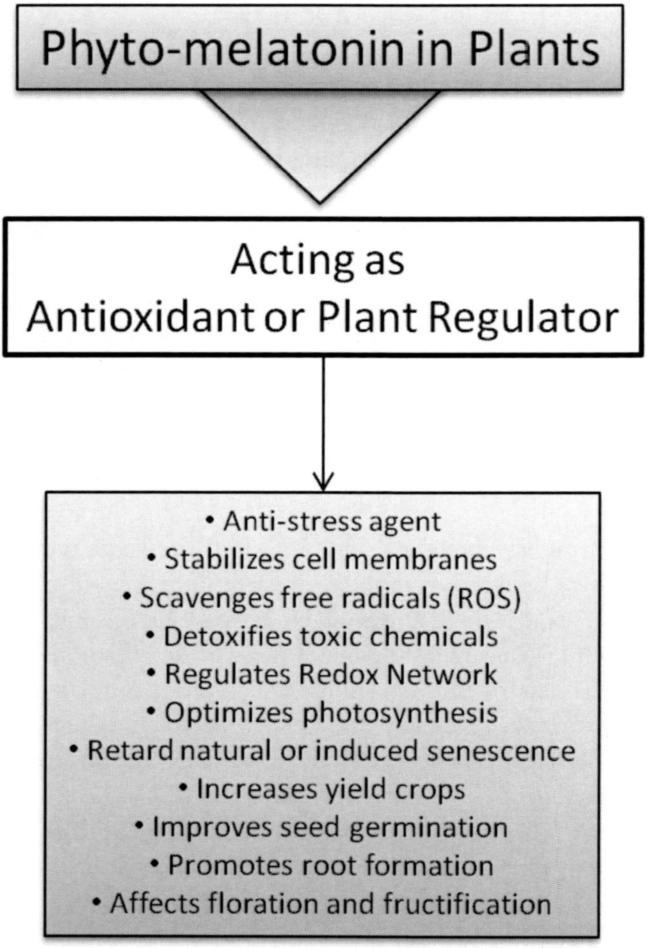

Figure 2. Possible roles of phyto-melatonin in higher plants.

3. Overview of Melatonin in Humans

Melatonin is known to act as a biological modulator of mood, sleep, body temperature, locomotor activity, food-intake, retina physiology, sexual behaviour, seasonal reproductive physiology, circadian rhythms and immunological enhancement (Figure 3) [10]. In mammals, melatonin is secreted from the pineal gland at night, from where it diffuses into the cerebrospinal fluid (CSF) and the blood stream, although levels quickly drop during the day. Thus, a role in photoperiodic regulation has been demonstrated because of the duration and timing of the melatonin signal [55-58]. Another important action attributed to melatonin is its scavenging capacity against biological free radicals (antioxidant activity), such as reactive oxygen species (ROS) and reactive nitrogen species (RNS) including hydroxyl radical, singlet oxygen, peroxyl radical, hydrogen peroxide, peroxynitrite anion and nitric oxide. In this way it protects cells and tissues from oxidative stress.

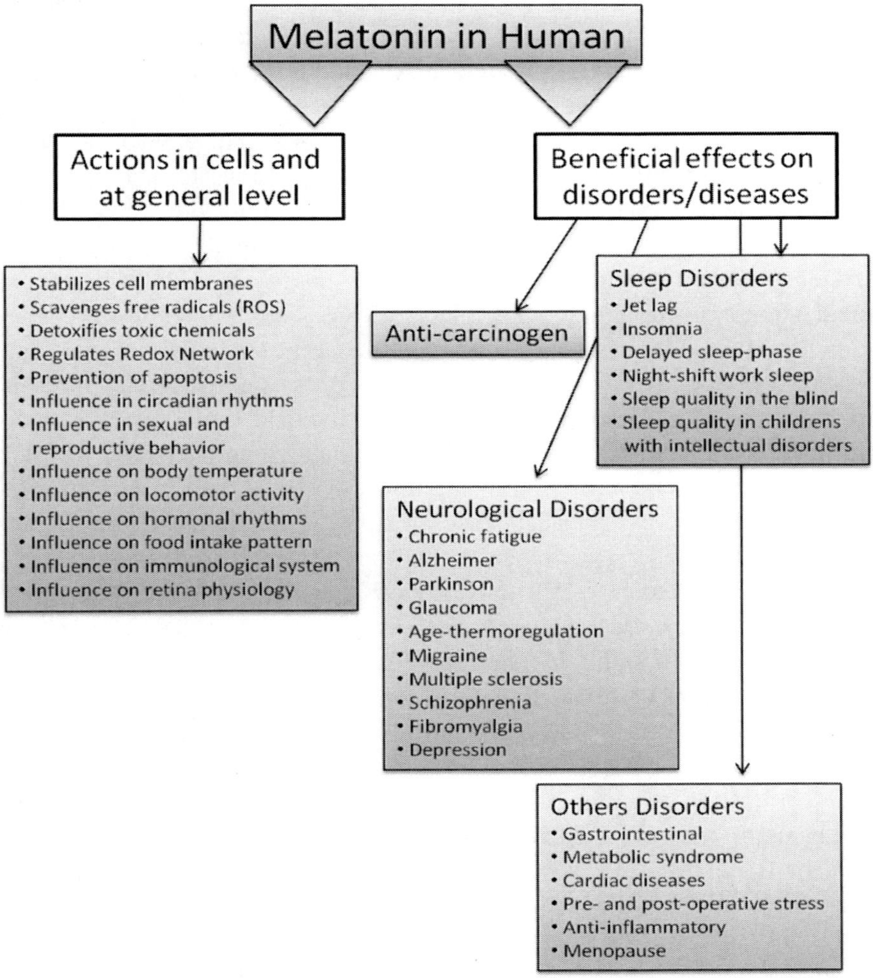

Figure 3. Roles of melatonin in human.

In humans, melatonin is well known for its role as a chronobiological agent, acting as an endogenous synchronizer of endocrine rhythms. Melatonin regulates sleep-wake cycles through a 'darkness signal,' whereby it alerts the brain and peripheral organs. Melatonin is a sleep initiator which opens the circadian sleep-gate. It adjusts the timing and reinforces the oscillations of the biological clock. The signal appears during the night because melatonin is secreted by the pineal gland into the cerebrospinal liquid (CSF) and released into the bloodstream. Melatonin levels reach a maximum in the middle of the night. Brief exposure to light provokes a decrease in melatonin biosynthesis. The circadian pattern of melatonin secretion is regulated by the biological clock of the hypothalamic suprachiasmatic nucleus (SCN), which is synchronized to changes in environmental light detected by the retina. Melatonin production by the pineal gland continues until the age of twenty, after which it declines with age. Melatonin oscillations also regulate vital activity related with seasonal periods and reproductive functions [59-62].

Exogenous melatonin administration alters the timing of body rhythms, including sleep, where phase delays are observed with the morning administration of melatonin, while phase advances are found after its evening administration. Many sleep disorders have been treated with melatonin: delayed sleep phase syndrome, night shift-work sleep disorder, seasonal affective disorder, sleep disorders in the blind and aging, and in patho-physiological disorders of children, with notable improvements in 'sleep quality' [63-68]. The most widespread disorder treated with melatonin is jet-lag, a de-phasing in the sleep-wake rhythms resulting from trans-oceanic flights [69] (Figure 3). Neurological and other disorders have been related to alterations in melatonin oscillations or their receptors, including Alzheimer's and Parkinson's syndrome, glaucoma and macular degeneration, syndrome of chronic fatigue, multiple sclerosis, depression, schizophrenia, anxiety, menopause, gastrointestinal disease, coronary disease and cardiac diseases, changes in food intake patterns related with obesity, osteoporosis and as geroprotector. The possible link of melatonin with cancer has been associated with its function as down-regulator of the pituitary and gonadal hormones which control mammary gland development, among other factors. These same indications regarding the effect of alterations in the sleep-wake cycle and cancer risk have been studied in connection with the proliferation of colorectal cancer in female nurses. Complementary to all these actions, melatonin is an immunomodulator capable of activating lymphocytes and monocytes/macrophages, and, by means of immunosurveillance, cancer cells can be detected and eliminated, preventing tumor development (see more cites in [10]).

4. Possible Effects of Phyto-Melatonin in Human Health

The intake of 'natural products' in a balanced diet is considered a contributor to human health. While nutritional supplements are many and various, dietitians and nutritionists are increasingly recommending the consumption of natural foods with proven health-promoting effects, such as fruits, vegetables, cereals, nuts, vegetal oils and beneficial herbs, among others. Thus, the intake of phyto-melatonin could be correlated with the consumption of plant foodstuffs. As mentioned above, phyto-melatonin from plant foods is absorbed from the gastrointestinal tract, modulating blood melatonin levels. Melatonin has a short average life in the blood, around 20-40 min, after which its level in blood decay as a result of the body's metabolism and its elimination in urine [70-72].

The scientific literature contains several examples of the effect that phyto-melatonin absorption has or could have on human health. Besides studies in animals, some data exists for humans. As examples we can cite as follows:

Example 1

In rats fed walnuts [35] and in chicks fed grains [3], an increase in serum circulating phyto-melatonin can be observed. In these cases, the intake of phyto-melatonin-rich plants produces a net increase (up to 4-fold the basal level) in melatonin levels in the bloodstream. This increase occurs 60-120 min after the consumption of phyto-melatonin-rich plants. In the case of rats fed walnuts, a correlated increase in antioxidant activity in blood was observed, indicating that phyto-melatonin (and also other phyto-substances) improves the antioxidant-pool.

Example 2

Similarly, in humans, the same effect has been found. Thus, the consumption of sweet cherries (prepared as a powdered freeze-dried product) caused a notable rise of 6-sulfatoxymelatonin (the main urinary degradation metabolite of melatonin in humans), in young, middle-aged, and elderly subjects. Also, a direct correlation with the antioxidant capacity was observed.

The studies demonstrate that many sleep-quality parameters such as sleep efficiency, actual sleep time, total nocturnal activity and immobility, can be improved [73, 74].

Example 3

Healthy volunteers who drank one or two beers (330 or 660 mL) showed a clear increase in blood melatonin levels compared with basal melatonin levels, 45 min after drinking. Similarly, an increase in blood antioxidant levels in the group that drank beer was observed. This effect can be related to the antioxidants available in beer, such as organic acids, vitamin B, silicic acid and flavonoids. One of the conclusions reached is that the phyto-melatonin in beer may protect the body from oxidative stress damage due to its excellent antioxidant properties [75].

Example 4

In another cross-over trial, serum melatonin levels increased 120 min after tropical fruit consumption. Although the tropical fruits assayed (orange, pineapple and banana) have moderate or low phyto-melatonin levels, consumption clearly produces a rise in human serum melatonin levels (up to 5-fold the basal level) [22, 24]. This, together with their antioxidant capacity, suggests that any type of fruit or plant extract, even with low levels of phyto-melatonin, can influence blood melatonin levels.

The most relevant aspects where the intake of phyto-melatonin-rich plants might have an effect are following described:

4.1. Phyto-Melatonin Acting as Antioxidant

The excellent qualities of melatonin as an antioxidant, mentioned above, will be significantly enhanced in the case of phyto-melatonin. In this respect, it is interesting to note that melatonin shows certain peculiarities as an antioxidant: *i)* the melatonin molecule presents no pro-oxidative effects, *ii)* melatonin-intermediate products also show antioxidant properties and *iii)* melatonin shows an important synergistic action with other antioxidants, such as ascorbic acid, glutathione, *etc*. In the case of phyto-melatonin, as a naturally occurring substance always obtained from natural plant extracts (without external contamination or additions), it goes hand in hand with many other hydrophilic natural compounds, such as organic acids (vitamin C), phenolic acids, flavonoids and anthocyanins. In some cases, it can also be accompanied by carotenoids (provitamin A) or tocopherols (vitamin E), compounds of a lipophilic nature. The presence of these compounds with phyto-melatonin can enhance its antioxidant properties through synergistic actions [76-79].

Recent data clearly indicate that increases in phyto-melatonin in the blood are accompanied by increases in serum antioxidant capacity (as can be seen in the above Examples) [71, 80]. This combination (phyto-melatonin together with various plant antioxidants) has no harmful effects, like the pro-oxidant activity that is found in many synthetic vitamin supplements. Related to the antioxidant activity of melatonin, are multiple beneficial health effects in combating diseases and disorders related to oxidative stress and cellular aging (see above).

4.2. Phyto-Melatonin Acting as Anti-Cancerigen

Melatonin can act as an anticancerigenic and antitumoral agent. This interesting effect has been studied in multiple cancer types such as breast, lung, liver, renal, pancreatic, colo-rectal, testicular, endometrial, cervico-vaginal, skin, brain and lymphoma. The action of melatonin on cancer cells has been related with its ability to reduce DNA damage, the up-regulation of antioxidative enzymes, changes in the expression of growth- and differentiation-related genes, reduction of some mitogenic signals, reduction of the metastatic capacity of tumor cells through the control of some oncogenesis-related genes, among others. In some cases, many cancers have been associated with low melatonin levels in serum or with deficiencies of melatonin-receptors in damaged tissues. Some therapies use melatonin to stop tumor proliferation [1, 80-88].

4.3. Phyto-Melatonin Acting as Gastrointestinal Tract Protector

Melatonin can also be produced by human organs other than the pineal gland. This so-called "extra-pineal melatonin" is generated by many different tissues/cells, such as the gastrointestinal tract, retina, several leukocytes, bone marrow, cerebral cortex, liver, thymus, spleen, heart, muscle, placenta, testis and skin [89-92]. In quantitative terms, extra-pineal melatonin is a hundred-times more plentiful than that generated in the pineal gland, but it seems to be only released into the bloodstream for very short time periods. However, it has been noted that large amounts of melatonin from the gastrointestinal tract enter the blood during the post-prandial response. Food intake results in an increase in the plasma concentration of melatonin (see above Examples). These pulses of melatonin seem to have little effect on the circadian system for their brevity and the fact that they occur in the silent point of the phase response curve. Gastrointestinal melatonin prevents ulceration of the gastro-intestinal mucosa, reduces hydrochloric acid secretion, stimulates the immunological system, increases micro-circulation and promotes epithelial regeneration, among other actions [93-96].

4.4. Phyto-Melatonin Acting As Sleep-Quality Enhancer and Jet-Lag Remedy

Another aspect of interest is that phyto-melatonin-rich plants may be responsible for a sleep-inducing effect due to its known role in circadian rhythms, especially in sleep quality (see Example 2). Melatonin blood plasma concentration is basically very low: below 0.01 nanograms per mL, during the day and around 0.2 nanograms per mL maximum at night [96]. Taking into account the phyto-melatonin levels in some plants (see Tables 1-6), an uptake of bloodstream-bound phyto-melatonin from plant foods might be expected (see Examples 1-4). It has also been suggested that the high levels of phyto-melatonin in plants act as a compensatory mechanism for animals. The limited data that exist indicate that consuming plant foodstuffs containing phyto-melatonin alters circulating levels of the same and increases 6-sulfatoxymelatonin (a direct catabolite) concentrations in the urine (see Examples 2 and 4) [97]. This may have implications as regards its sleep-enhancing effect, improving sleep and certain pathological conditions associated with sleep such as insomnia, among others (see previous section). Indeed, age-related disturbances in the sleep–wake and temperature rhythms have been correlated with age-related reductions in the amplitude of the nocturnal melatonin peak. In fact, the loss of melatonin in advanced age leads to disturbances of the circadian pacemaker, which causes internal temporal desynchronization in the central and peripheral clocks, inducing a variety of chronopathologies and leading to the generalized deterioration of health. Thus, the consumption of plant foodstuffs may be beneficial as they may enhance the health effects mediated by phyto-melatonin against sleep disorders. Also, the ingestion of phyto-melatonin-rich foods could be involved in post-prandial sleepiness [63, 68, 98-100].

The intake of melatonin pills to attenuate jet lag is widespread [101-103], and, although to a lesser extent, the consumption of melatonin as a geroprotective agent seems to have many followers [67, 104]. In this sense, it has been seen that the oral administration of melatonin at 1–300 mg, or up to 1 g daily for 30 days had no adverse side effects, although in some cases somnolence and headache were described as symptoms [105-107].

Generally, in patients subject to sleep disturbance (due to age or other causes), it is recommended that melatonin pills at different doses be taken at the end of the afternoon, a few hours before bedtime. This time often coincides with the end of dinner, providing an accumulative effect with post-prandial melatonin (from food), and the natural rise in pineal melatonin in the blood. All this means that in some patients, melatonin levels may be too high in the first few hours of sleep. Therefore, more studies are needed on the real contribution of phyto-melatonin in the bloodstream in these critical hours before bedtime. Given the wide variation in the pharmacokinetics of oral melatonin in humans, more studies are necessary to improve knowledge about its pharmacological profile: e.g., the pharmacodynamics of phyto-melatonin in healthy volunteers using different doses, times of administration, periods of treatment and quantitative contribution of phyto-melatonin through foods.

5. Differences Between Synthetic, Animal and Phyto-melatonin

Structurally, both melatonin and phyto-melatonin are the same molecule. As mentioned above, "melatonin" refers to melatonin of synthetic or animal origin and "phyto-melatonin" to that which has a plant origin.

Practically all the melatonin supplements that are marketed are made from synthetic melatonin. Previously, melatonin was obtained from animal sources such as cow or rats, but due to the risk of virus infection, synthetic production is often more common, in a process that is chemically simple and very productive [108-110].

There are various methods involving several synthetic organic routes, such as:

- Route 1.- From 5-methoxyindole-acetonitrile
- Route 2.- From 5-methoxynitroethylated indoles
- Route 3.- From 5-methoxytryptamine
- Route 4.- From phthalimide derivates

Since the discovery of melatonin in 1958 by Lerner and collaborators, its organic synthesis has been significantly improved, with more productive and economic processes. Route 3 and 4 appear to be the most feasible and commercially viable. Synthetic melatonin is generated at high yields (over 80%), while a whole series of residual compounds (chemical contaminants of the melatonin preparation processes) also appear. Table 7 shows some of the most common contaminants present in the synthetic melatonin preparations commercially available. Most occur at concentrations below 0.5% (relative to the amount of melatonin).

Table 7. Common contaminants in synthetic melatonin preparations

Contaminant compounds
1,2,3,4-tetrahydro-β-carboline-3-carboxylic acid
3-(phenylamino) alanine
1,1'-ethylidenebis(tryptophan)(peak E)
2-(3-indolylmethyl)-tryptophan
formaldehyde-melatonin
formaldehyde-melatonin condensation products
hydroxymelatonin isomers
1,3-diphthalimidopropane
hydroxy-bromo-propylphthalimide
chloropropylphthalimide
5-hydroxy-tryptamine derivatives
5-methoxy-tryptamine derivatives
N-acetyl and diacetyl indole derivatives

These melatonin-contaminants can be classified according the synthesis route used [111, 112]:

- In "classical" organic melatonin synthesis from methoxyindoles (Routes 1, 2 and 3), the above contaminants are related with the tryptophan molecule, and have also been described in tryptophan supplements as is shows in Table 7. Other contaminants such as oxidized forms of melatonin or condensation-related products, arise from the instability of the melatonin molecule.

- In Route 4, several specific melatonin contaminants, all derived from phthalimide, may appear. Up to 14 different contaminants have been described in the process of organic synthesis of melatonin from phthalamide, some of which are listed in Table 7.

Eosinophilia-myalgia syndrome (EMS), an incurable and sometimes fatal disease (by mid-1990 there had been 27 deaths associated to EMS, but only a single case in 2011), has been related to the presence of L-tryptophan-derivatives (up to 60 contaminants) in some poorly produced-tryptophan dietary supplements (mainly the so-called "peak E" listed in Table 7). In the case of melatonin supplements, the ingestion of these contaminants is much lower because the daily dosage recommended of melatonin are up to a thousand times lower than the recommended for L-tryptophan supplements [113, 114]. As regards to phthalimide, this widely used chemical is currently subject to multiple toxicological investigations [115]. Curiously, despite the many years that it has been studied, there are no conclusive data. Although the fact that this molecule is present in toxic compounds such as pesticides and fungicides, among others, suggests that some degree of toxicity is expected. Only irritability of the eyes, dermatitis through skin contact and respiratory tract sensitization has been officially notified: *"Chronic Potential Health Effects: no information found at this time. The toxicological properties of this substance have not been fully investigated."* Some studies on possible teratogenic, mutagenic and genotoxic effects due to the similarity with thalidomide and fungicides (folpet, captan) have been suggested. In either case, there is a very small degree of risk involved in taking chemically synthesized melatonin supplements. Also, in some cases it has been claimed that synthetic melatonin does not exert the same effects as pineal melatonin, possibly due to errors in the amounts of melatonin supplied by the manufacturer or through incorrect dosage.

In the case of phyto-melatonin, its *a priori* natural origin should rule out any possibility of chemical contamination. Not only that, but the phyto-melatonin obtained from plant extracts are "accompanied" by a set of other natural substances including antioxidants, vitamins, simple phenols, flavonoids, carotenoids, tocopherols, among others. These compounds will co-participate in the beneficial functions that phyto-melatonin has in our body.

However, there is still some risk if phyto-melatonin formulations are not been obtained properly. The presence of solvent residues due to extraction protocols is common. Also, the plant source used must be controlled to avoid the presence of pesticides or other chemical compounds due to previous cultured or postharvest treatments. The use of wild plants or organically grown plants as source of phyto-melatonin should avoid the presence of undesirable chemicals in supplements. For extraction, it is advisable to use supercritical fluid extraction (SFE), using carbon dioxide (CO_2) at high pressure as harmless extractant. CO_2 is a good extraction solvent as it is chemically pure, non-toxic, non-flammable, non-polar, stable, colourless, odourless and tasteless. Importantly, it is easily removed and highly selective. Industrially, CO_2 is used in the beverage, food, flavour and cosmetics industries, partially because significant value is added to products that are processed using CO_2, since they can be labelled as environmental friendly. The application of *"Green Chemistry Principles"* with the use of alternative solvents, ensuring minimal contamination, could be a highly recommended practice for this type of supplement [116].

In some cases, phyto-melatonin has been obtained from plant extracts but using L-tryptophan as precursor in bioreactors [117]. The use of synthetic L-tryptophan leads to the situation described above, where a large amount of contaminants derived from L-tryptophan may appear in the formulations of an "*apparently natural*" phyto-melatonin. The only way to ensure the natural source of phyto-melatonin supplements is through rigorous control of their origin (plant species and cultivation mode) and of the reagents and extraction processes employed. The presence of well known "*contaminants derived from L-tryptophan*" will give us a clear clue to the unnatural origin. The great problem is that the detection and identification of these contaminants requires very sophisticated techniques such as liquid chromatography mass spectrometry (LC-MS) or gas chromatography mass spectrometry (GC-MS), in its multiple possibilities.

6. Availability of Melatonin and Phyto-Melatonin Supplements

Dietary supplement and food supplement are foods whose objective is to supplement the diet. They consist of concentrated nutrients or substances that have some physiological effect. These food supplements are a growing market in both developed and developing countries. Some factors that make them interesting are their affordable prices, their availability without medied prescription and the perception (through marketing) that they are natural and safe products. The legislation of such supplements differs in the European Union (EU)[1] and USA[2].

The EU includes them in the same regulations as those refering to foods, while there is a specified regulation for dietary supplements in the USA. The official agency, the Food and Drug Administration (FDA) do not subject these products to control or evaluation (nor as regards their composition or doses), but requires that *"these statements have not been evaluated by the FDA"* appear on the label[3]. In the case of the EU and exclusively with respect to melatonin, two health claims for food containing melatonin have been authorized[4,5]:

- *"helps relieve the subjective feeling of jet-lag,"* which requires a minimum daily intake of 0.5 mg and
- *"helps reduce the time required to fall asleep,"* which requires a minimum daily intake of 1 mg.

As mentioned above, practically all the melatonin supplements that are marketed are made from synthetic melatonin. Simple and composite formulations are constituted by synthetic melatonin in a very wide range of forms such as tablets, pills, sublingual, liquids, gels, creams; even suppositories, and at different dosage (from 0.1 mg to 400 mg). In the case of composite formulations, synthetic melatonin is presented together with other

---

[1] Regulation (EC) no 178/2002 of the European Parlament and of the Council laying down the general principles and requirements of food law, establishing the European Food Safety Authority and laying down procedures in matters of food safety. *Official Journal of the European Communities* L31, 1–24, 2002.

[2] Dietary Supplement Health and Education Act of 1994. *Public Law 103-417. 103rd Congress.* Stat 4325 (codified at 21 USC 301. 9).

[3] Guidance for Industry: Substantiation for Dietary Supplement Claims Made Under Section 403(r) (6) of the Federal Food, Drug, and Cosmetic Act. Food and Drug Administration, 2008; Guidance for Industry: FDA's Implementation of Qualified Health Claims": Questions and Answers; *Final Guidance. Food and Drug Administration*, 2006.

[4] Scientific Opinion on the substantiation of health claims related to melatonin and alleviation of subjective feelings of jet lag (ID 1953), and reduction of sleep onset latency, and improvement of sleep quality (ID 1953) pursuant to Article 13(1) of Regulation (EC) No 1924/20061 EFSA Panel on Dietetic Products, Nutrition and Allergies (NDA). *EFSA Journal* 2010, *8(2)*, 1467.

[5] Scientific Opinion on the substantiation of a health claim related to melatonin and reduction of sleep onset latency (ID 1698, 1780, 4080) pursuant to Article 13(1) of Regulation (EC) No 1924/20061 EFSA Panel on Dietetic Products, Nutrition and Allergies (NDA). *EFSA Journal* 2011, *9(6)*, 2241.

compounds (generally also synthetic) such as tryptophan, vitamins (C, B6), minerals; even collagen, and hyaluronic acid, in the case of creams.

Lastly, some particular preparations are available. These are formulations that combine synthetic melatonin with medicinal plants. These are bi-layer tablets, with synthetic melatonin (fast action) and plant extracts (slow action). The plants used in this type of mixed formulation (Table 8) reveal some pharmacological effects such as relaxing, calmative or sedative activities.

Although much remains to be investigated, many phytochemical and pharmacological data of the plants described exist. In most cases, the data refer to alkaloids, terpenoids (mono-, sesquiterpenoids, iridoids, *etc.*), phenolic acids and isoflavonoids and flavonoids (anthoxanthins (flavones and flavonols), flavanones, flavanonols, flavans and anthocyanidins)), as agents related to the relaxing and sleep promoting properties. Interestingly, no mention is made of the possible presence of phyto-melatonin in these plant extracts, possibly due to the novel aspect of phyto-melatonin, although its presence has been demonstrated in some of the most common medicinal plants. This is surprising, since the presence of phyto-melatonin in medicinal plants was demonstrated in 1995, but curiously, no data of phyto-melatonin content in plants used as sleeping aids (as the above cited) have been published.

Only some data on the phyto-melatonin content of related species are available (Table 9).

Table 8. Medicinal plants with sedative properties used in mixed formulations

Valerian (*Valeriana officinalis* L.)
Passionflower (*Passiflora incarnata* L.)
Scullcap (*Scutelaria galericulata* L./*S. lateriflora* L.)
Lemon balm (*Melissa officinalis* L.)
Linden (*Tilia platyphyllos* L.)
Californian poppy (*Eschscholzia californica* Cham.)
Aloe[1] (*Aloe vera* L.)
Lavender[1] (*Lavandula angustifolia*) Miller
Avocado[1] (*Persea americana* Miller)

[1]In the case of creams

Table 9. Phyto-melatonin content of some medicinal plants related with sleeping aids

Common Name/Species	Phyto-melatonin content
Scullcap (*Scutellaria amoena* C. H. Wright)	178 ng/g DW[1]
Hawthorn (*Crataegus sp.*)	0.3-0.43 ng/g FW[2]
Corn poppy (*Papaver rhoea* L.)	6 ng/g DW
Aloe (*Aloe vera* L.)	516 ng/g DW

[1]DW: dry weight; [2]FW: fresh weight

At present, only four formulations exclusively composed of phyto-melatonin are known. Even though the laboratories that market it do not give much information on its origin, it appears that in three cases synthetic melatonin is not used in the formulation. Some characteristics of these formulations with phyto-melatonin are presented in the following Table 10.

Table 10. Different commercial formulations containing phyto-melatonin

	Trademark	Origin	Dosis	Form (units)	Brand
#1	HerbatoninPRO	Rice extract	0.3 mg	Capsules (120)	Natural Health International USA
#2	Sleep Support	Tart cherry skins Tart cherry juice	15 μg 3 μg	Capsules (60) Sachets (liquid)	Tru2U New Zeland
#3	Melatonin 10 mg	Vegetarian	10 mg	Sublingual tablets (180)	Bioclinic Naturals Canada
#4	Curaderm system	Multiple plants	?	Cream	Curapharm USA

Some comments about these formulations can be made.

a) In the case of **Formulation #1** (in Table 10), the information is scant. It is unknown whether the source of the phyto-melatonin is entire rice plants, rice grains (seeds) or waste products of the rice plant. We know that the contents of phyto-melatonin in rice plants (Table 11) are.

Table 11. Phyto-melatonin content in rice plant organs

Rice Plant Organ	Seed/grain	Stem	Leaf	Flower	Root
Phyto-melatonin content (ng/g FW)	1	0.5	0.1	0.4	0.2

Thus, taking into account the amount of phyto-melatonin in rice seeds, to obtain only one capsule with 0.3 mg of phyto-melatonin, 300 kg (661 lb) of rice grains would need to be processed; this represents 36,000 kg (79,366 lb) of rice per package …Surprising!

b) Formulation #2 (in Table 10) is the only one that indicates exactly the source of phyto-melatonin: freeze-dried Montmorency tart cherry skin extract, and also juice. In this case, we also know the content of tart cherries, a mean value of 14 ng of phyto-melatonin/g fruit (without seed) (see Table 1). To obtain one capsule (15 micrograms, 1μg = 10^{-6} gram = 0.001 mg) of phyto-melatonin, according to the manufacturer, about 1 kg (2.2 lb) of cherries would be necessary; this represents 64 kg (141 lb) of cherries per package. This represents credible data.

c) Formulation #3 (in Table 10) provides least information, since it merely says that the phyto-melatonin comes from *"vegetarian source."* Surprisingly, each tablet contains 10 mg of phyto-melatonin! It is impossible to calculate the tons of plant material needed to produce just one package with these phyto-melatonin capsules.

d) Formulation #4 (in Table 10) is an anti-aging skin cream composed of a blend of selected botanical herbs that *"…contain full spectrum antioxidants … for healthier hair skin and nails,"* according to the label. In the information given, the company is committed to phyto-melatonin (all natural) *versus* synthetic melatonin (with multiple chemical contaminants). The product contains the following plants: Chinese Angelica (Danghui), *Lycium* fruit (Goji berry), Jujube, Scullcap, Ginseng, Chinese licorice root (*Glycyrrhiza uralensis*), Chinese foxglove (*Rehmania chinensis*), Squisandra (*Schizandra chinensis*), among other ingredients (aloe, milk-vetch, cinnamon bark, manuka honey, *etc.*). Practically all the above herbs contain high level of phyto-melatonin, but, since we do not known the relative amount of each plant, the amount or concentration of phyto-melatonin in this preparation cannot be calculated.

Based on Tables 1-6, the plant material used in Formulations #1, #2 and #3 do not seem to have been rigorously selected, since other sources contain much higher phyto-melatonin levels, as is the case of many medicinal plants (Formulation #4) (Table 6). Surely, manufacturers must begin to consider these data. In many cases, the raw material is often a decisive factor in production costs. The use of plant by-products or waste from agricultural or food industry is often a common practice in order to lower the production costs. In the case of phyto-melatonin supplements, choosing low cost raw material should take into account the levels of endogenous phyto-melatonin in the plant material selected. The choice of raw materials with low levels of phyto-melatonin entails processing vast amounts of plant material to obtain minimal quantities of the product of interest.

7. Quality Controls Are Necessary

Currently, neither EU nor USA legislation requires analytical checks on these dietary/food supplements. Nor does the information provided by the manufacturers seem sufficient, so the consumer is faced with a difficult situation from the point of view of really knowing the characteristics of the product that they are consuming. Total security that the purchased product contains 100% natural substances can only come if exhaustive analyses, to exclude the presence of L-tryptophan contaminants are performed. Even with a base or matrix of plant origin, the addition of synthetic substances, including melatonin and/or some of its metabolic precursors could also occur. In this scenario, it seems that the consumer can only rely on the responsibility and trust of the manufacturer, because official agencies rule out their liability. Clearly, we need more controls and the introduction of compulsory, thorough analysis that leave no doubt about the natural (or not) origin of these types of supplements. Also, the ability to contrast general information and particular data on plant sources will enable the consumer to select which products to buy. Indeed, this hope is the driving force behind this book chapter.

Conclusion

- The presence of phyto-melatonin in all plant species analyzed has opened the door to its use as a natural nutraceutical compound.
- Aromatic and medicinal plants present significantly higher phyto-melatonin levels than seeds and fleshy fruits. Such herbs are the best candidates for shaping the future melatonin supplements.
- The search and study of phyto-melatonin-rich species and varieties should take priority.
- The control of growth conditions might help us to obtain phyto-melatonin-rich plants. More studies in more plants and varieties are necessary.

- Phyto-melatonin has a great potential as a therapy for many diseases both at physiological and pharmacological doses.
- Its antioxidant, anticancerigen, and rhythm-synchronizing properties (sleep-promoting properties), among others, are an excellent area in which its use as nutraceutical could have wide beneficial applications.
- The absence of undesirable substances (contaminants generated during the chemical synthesis of melatonin) is the key factor in choosing phyto-melatonin as a "100% natural" supplement.
- It is best to consume fresh natural products with high melatonin levels to improve sleep quality when some related disorders appear.
- New preparations containing phyto-melatonin will inevitably appear. Surely, a turnaround in the marketing of melatonin supplements is due, synthetic supplements being displaced by natural substances such as phyto-melatonin.
- It is to be hoped that such products will contain natural substances whose origin and possible contamination will be strictly controlled.
- I hope that in any subsequent edition of this book I will be able to describe many more preparations based on phyto-melatonin, and to further discuss botanical and pharmacological aspects.

REFERENCES

[1] Blask DE, Dauchy RT, Sauer LA, Krause JA. Melatonin uptake and growth prevention in rat hepatoma 7288CTC in response to dietary melatonin: melatonin receptor-mediated inhibition of tumor linoleic acid metabolism to the growth signaling molecule 13-hydroxyoctadecadienoic acid and the potential role of phytomelatonin. *Carcinogenesis* 25(6), 951-960, 2004.

[2] Dubbels R, Reiter RJ, Klenke E, Goebel A, Schnakenberg E, Ehlers C, Schiwara HW, Schloot W. Melatonin in edible plants identified by radioimmunoassay and by HPLC-MS. *J Pineal Res* 18(1), 28-31, 1995.

[3] Hattori A, Migitaka H, Iigo M, Yamamoto K, Ohtani-Kaneko R, Hara M, Suzuki T, Reiter RJ. Identification of melatonin in plants and its effects on plasma melatonin levels and binding to melatonin receptors in vertebrates. *Biochem Mol Biol Int* 35(3), 627-634, 1995.

[4] Lerner AB, Case JD, Takahashi Y, Lee TH, Mori W. Isolation of melatonin, a pineal factor that lightens melanocytes. *J Am Chem Soc* 80(10), 2587, 1958.

[5] Lerner A, Case J, Mori W, Wright M. Melatonin in peripheral nerve. *Nature* 183, 1821, 1959.

[6] Vivien-Roels B, Pévet P, Beck O, Fevre-Montange M. Identification of melatonin in the compound eyes of an insect, the locust *(Locusta migratoria)* by radioimmunoassay and gas chromatography-mass spectrometry. *Neurosci Lett* 49(1-2), 153-157, 1984.

[7] Morita M, Hall F, Best JB, Gern W. Photoperiodic modulation of cephalic melatonin in planarians. *J Exp Zool* 241(3), 383-388, 1987.

[8] Callebert J, Jaunay JM, Jallon JM. Control of *Drosophilla* biorhythms. *Adv Pineal Res* 5, 81-84, 1991.

[9] Arnao MB, Hernández-Ruiz J. The physiological function of melatonin in plants. *Plant Sign Behav* 1(1), 89-95, 2006.

[10] Arnao MB, Hernández-Ruiz J. (Chapter 21) Melatonin: Synthesis From Tryptophan and Its Role in Higher Plants. pp 390-435. In: D' Mello J (ed) *Amino Acids in Higher Plants*. 2015 (published). Boston, USA, CAB Intern.

[11] Arnao MB, Hernández-Ruiz J. Functions of melatonin in plants: a review. *J Pineal Res* 59(2), 133-150, 2015.

[12] Potterat O. Goji (*Lycium barbarum and L-chinense*): phytochemistry, pharmacology and safety in the perspective of traditional uses and recent popularity. *Planta Medica* 76(1), 7-19, 2010.

[13] Ramakrishna A, Giridhar P, Sankar K, Ravishankar G. Melatonin and serotonin profiles in beans of *Coffea* species. *J Pineal Res* 52(4), 470-476, 2012.

[14] Chen G, Huo Y, Tan DX, Liang Z, Zhang W, Zhang Y. Melatonin in chinese medicinal herbs. *Life Sci* 73(1), 19-26, 2003.

[15] Lei Q, Wang L, Tan DX, Zhao Y, Zheng XD, Chen H, Li Qt, Zuo Bx, Kong J. Identification of genes for melatonin synthetic enzymes in Red Fuji apple (*Malus domestica* Borkh.cv.Red) and their expression and melatonin production during fruit development. *J Pineal Res* 55(4), 443-451, 2013.

[16] Zhao Y, Tan DX, Lei Q, Chen H, Wang L, Li Qt, Gao Y, Kong J. Melatonin and its potential biological functions in the fruits of sweet cherry. *J Pineal Res* 55(1), 79-88, 2013.

[17] Burkhardt S, Tan DX, Manchester LC, Hardeland R, Reiter RJ. Detection and quantification of the antioxidant melatonin in montmorency and balaton tart cherries (*Prunus cerasus*). *J Agr Food Chem* 49(10), 4898-4902, 2001.

[18] Vitalini S, Gardana C, Zanzotto A, Simonetti P, Faoro F, Fico G, Iriti M. The presence of melatonin in grapevine (*Vitis vinifera* L.) berry tissues. *J Pineal Res* 51(3), 331-337, 2011.

[19] Mena P, Gil-Izquierdo A, Moreno DA, Martí N, García-Viguera C. Assessment of the melatonin production in pomegranate wines. *LWT Food Sci Technol* 47(1), 13-18, 2012.

[20] Zohar R, Izhaki I, Koplovich A, Ben-Shlomo R. Phytomelatonin in the leaves and fruits of wild perennial plants. *Phytochem Lett* 4(3), 222-226, 2011.

[21] Fernández-Pachón MS, Medina S, Herrero-Martín G, Cerrillo I, Berná G, Escudero-López B, Ferreres F, Martín F, García-Parrilla MC, Gil-Izquierdo A. Alcoholic fermentation induces melatonin synthesis in orange juice. *J Pineal Res* 56(1), 31-38, 2014.

[22] Johns NP, Johns J, Porasupthana S, Plaimee P, Sae-Teaw M. Dietary intake of melatonin from tropical fruit altered urinary excretion of 6-sulfatoxymelatonin in healthy volunteers. *J Agr Food Chem* 61(4), 913-919, 2013.

[23] Badria F. Melatonin, serotonin, tryptamine in some egyptian food and medicinal plants. *J Med Food* 5(3), 153-157, 2002.

[24] Sae-Teaw M, Johns J, Johns NP, Subongkot S. Serum melatonin levels and antioxidant capacities after consumption of pineapple, orange, or banana by healthy male volunteers. *J Pineal Res* 55(1), 58-64, 2013.

[25] Sturtz M, Cerezo A, Cantos-Villar E, Garcia-Parrilla M. Determination of the melatonin content of different varieties of tomatoes (*Lycopersicon esculentum*) and strawberries (*Fragaria ananassa*). *Food Chem* 127(3), 1329-1334, 2011.

[26] Huang X, Mazza G. Simultaneous analysis of serotonin, melatonin, piceid and resveratrol in fruits using liquid chromatography tandem mass spectrometry. *J Chromatogr A* 1218(25), 3890-3899, 2011.

[27] Pasko P, Sulkowska-Ziaja K, Muszynska B, Zagrodzki P. Serotonin, melatonin, and certain indole derivatives profiles in rutabaga and kohlrabi seeds, sprouts, bulbs, and roots. *LWT Food Sci Technol* 59(2), 740-745, 2014.

[28] Hernández-Ruiz J, Cano A, Arnao MB. Melatonin acts as a growth-stimulating compound in some monocot species. *J Pineal Res* 39(2), 137-142, 2005.

[29] Hernández-Ruiz J, Arnao MB. Distribution of melatonin in different zones of lupin and barley plants at different ages in the presence and absence of light. *J Agr Food Chem* 56(22), 10567-10573, 2008.

[30] Kocadagh T, Yilmaz C, Gokmen V. Determination of melatonin and its isomer in foods by liquid chromatography tandem mass spectrometry. *Food Chem* 153, 151-156, 2014.

[31] Pothinuch P, Tongchitpakdee S. Melatonin contents in mulberry (*Morus* spp.) leaves: Effects of sample preparation, cultivar, leaf age and tea processing. *Food Chem* 128(2), 415-419, 2011.

[32] Rodriguez-Naranjo M, Gil-Izquierdo A, Troncoso A, Cantos E, Garcia-Parrilla M. Melatonin: A new bioactive compound in wine. *J Food Comp Anal* 24, 603-608, 2011.

[33] Manchester LC, Tan DX, Reiter RJ, Park W, Monis K, Qi W. High levels of melatonin in the seeds of edible plants. Possible function in germ tissue protection. *Life Sci* 67(25), 3023-3029, 2000.

[34] Posmyk MM, Balabusta M, Wieczorek M, Sliwinska E, Janas KM. Melatonin applied to cucumber (*Cucumis sativus* L.) seeds improves germination during chilling stress. *J Pineal Res* 46(2), 214-223, 2009.

[35] Reiter R, Manchester L, Tan D. Melatonin in walnuts: influence on levels of melatonin and total antioxidant capacity of blood. *Nutrition* 21(9), 920-924, 2005.

[36] de la Puerta C, Carrascosa-Salmoral M, Garcia-Luna P, Lardone P, Herrera J, Fernandez-Montesinos R, Guerrero J, Pozo D. Melatonin is a phytochemical in olive oil. *Food Chem* 104(2), 609-612, 2007.

[37] Stege PW, Sombra LL, Messina G, Martinez LD, Silva MF. Determination of melatonin in wine and plant extracts by capillary electrochromatography with immobilized carboxylic multi-walled carbon nanotubes as stationary phase. *Electrophoresis* 31(13), 2242-2248, 2010.

[38] Afreen F, Zobayed SMA, Kozai T. Melatonin in *Glycyrrhiza uralensis*: response of plant roots to spectral quality of light and UV-B radiation. *J Pineal Res* 41(2), 108-115, 2006.

[39] Murch SJ, Saxena PK. A melatonin-rich germplasm line of St John's wort (*Hypericum perforatum* L.). *J Pineal Res* 41(3), 284-287, 2006.

[40] Murch SJ, Simmons CB, Saxena PK. Melatonin in feverfew and other medicinal plants. *Lancet* 350(9091), 1598-1599, 1997.

[41] Simopoulos AP, Tan DX, Manchester LC, Reiter RJ. Purslane: a plant source of omega-3 fatty acids and melatonin. *J Pineal Res* 39(3), 331-332, 2005.

[42] Arnao MB. Phytomelatonin: discovery, content, and role in plants. *Adv Bot* e815769, 2014.

[43] Arnao MB, Hernández-Ruiz J. Growth conditions influence the melatonin content of tomato plants. *Food Chem* 138, 1212-1214, 2013.

[44] Arnao MB, Hernández-Ruiz J. Melatonin: plant growth regulator and/or biostimulator during stress? *Trends Plant Sci* 19(12), 789-797, 2014.

[45] Arnao MB, Hernández-Ruiz J. Chemical stress by different agents affects the melatonin content of barley roots. *J Pineal Res* 46(3), 295-299, 2009.

[46] Arnao MB, Hernández-Ruiz J. Growth conditions determine different melatonin levels in *Lupinus albus* L. *J Pineal Res* 55(2), 149-155, 2013.

[47] Wang P, Sun X, Li C, Wei Z, Liang D, Ma F. Long-term exogenous application of melatonin delays drought-induced leaf senescence in apple. *J Pineal Res* 54(3), 292-302, 2013.

[48] Nawaz MA, Huang Y, Bie Z, Ahmad W, Reiter RJ, Niu M, Hameed S. Melatonin: current status and future perspectives in plant science. *Front Plant Sci* 6, 1230, 2016.

[49] Shi H, Chen K, Wei Y, He C. Fundamental issues of melatonin-mediated stress signaling in plants. *Front Plant Sci* 7, 1124, 2016.

[50] Shi H, Chen Y, Tan DX, Reiter RJ, Chan Z, He C. Melatonin induces nitric oxide and the potential mechanisms relate to innate immunity against bacterial pathogen infection in *Arabidopsis*. *J Pineal Res* 59(1), 102-108, 2015.

[51] Qian Y, Tan DX, Reiter RJ, Shi H. Comparative metabolomic analysis highlights the involvement of sugars and glycerol in melatonin-mediated innate immunity against bacterial pathogen in *Arabidopsis*. *Sci Rep* 5, 15815, 2015.

[52] Hernández-Ruiz J, Cano A, Arnao MB. Melatonin: growth-stimulating compound present in lupin tissues. *Planta* 220(1), 140-144, 2004.

[53] Arnao MB, Hernández-Ruiz J. Melatonin promotes adventitious- and lateral root regeneration in etiolated hypocotyls of *Lupinus albus* L. *J Pineal Res* 42(2), 147-152, 2007.

[54] Hernández-Ruiz J, Arnao MB. Phytomelatonin, an interesting tool for agricultural crops. *Focus Sci* 2(2), 1-7, 2016.

[55] Krause D, Dubocovich M. Regulatory sites in the melatonin system of mammals. *Trends Neurosci* 13(11), 464-470, 1990.

[56] Maronde E, Stehle JH. The mammalian pineal gland: known facts, unknown facets. *Trends Endocr Metabol* 18, 142-149, 2007.

[57] Gastel JA, Roseboom PH, Rinaldi PA, Weller JL, Klein DC. Melatonin production: proteasomal proteolysis in serotonin *N*-acetyltransferase regulation. *Science* 279(5355), 1358-1360, 1998.

[58] Jan JE, Reiter RJ, Wasdell MB, Bax M. The role of the thalamus in sleep, pineal melatonin production, and circadian rhythm sleep disorders. *J Pineal Res* 46(1), 1-7, 2009.

[59] Fuller PM, Gooley JJ, Saper CB. Neurobiology of the sleep-wake cycle: sleep architecture, circadian regulation, and regulatory feedback. *J Biol Rhythms* 21(6), 482-493, 2006.

[60] Saper CB, Scammell TE, Lu J. Hypothalamic regulation of sleep and circadian rhythms. *Nature* 437(7063), 1257-1263, 2005.

[61] Reiter RJ. The melatonin rhythm: both a clock and a calendar. *Experientia* 49(8), 654-664, 1993.

[62] Reppert SM, Weaver DR. Coordination of circadian timing in mammals. *Nature* 418(6901), 935-941, 2002.

[63] Claustrat B, Brun J, Chazot G. The basic physiology and pathophysiology of melatonin. *Sleep Medical Rev* 9(1), 11-24, 2005.

[64] Srinivasan V, Pandi-Perumal SR, Maestroni GJM, Esquifino AI, Hardeland R, Cardinali DP. Role of melatonin in neurodegenerative diseases. *Neurotoxicol Res* 7(4), 293-318, 2005.

[65] Witt-Enderby PA, Radio NM, Doctor JS, Davies VL. Therapeutics treatments potentially mediated by melatonin receptors: potential clinics uses in the prevention of osteoporosis, cancer and as an adjuvant therapy. *J Pineal Res* 41(4), 297-305, 2006.

[66] Wu YH, Swaab DF. The human pineal gland and melatonin in aging and Alzheimer's disease. *J Pineal Res* 38(3), 145-152, 2005.

[67] Hardeland R. Melatonin in aging and disease. Multiple consequences of reduced secretion, options and limits of treatment. *Aging Dis* 3(2), 194-225, 2012.

[68] Paredes S, Marchena A, Bejarano I, Espino J, Barriga C, Rial R, Reiter R, Rodriguez A. Melatonin and tryptophan affect the activity-rest rhythm, core and peripheral temperatures, and interleukin levels in the ringdove: changes with age. *J Gerontol Biol Sci* 64(3), 340-350, 2009.

[69] Waterhouse J, Reilly T, Atkinson G. Jet lag. *Lancet* 350(9091), 1611-1616, 1997.

[70] Korkmaz A, Reiter RJ, Tan DX, Manchester LC. Melatonin; from pineal gland to healthy foods. *Spatula DD* 1(1), 33-36, 2011.

[71] Reiter RJ, Tan DX, Burkhardt S, Manchester LC. Melatonin in plants. *Nutr Rev* 59(9), 286-290, 2001.

[72] Reiter RJ, Tan DX, Manchester LC, Simopoulos AP, Maldonado MD, Flores LJ, Terron MP. Melatonin in edible plants (phytomelatonin): identification, concentrations, bioavailability and proposed functions. *World Rev Nutr Diet* 97, 211-230, 2007.

[73] Garrido M, Espino J, González-Gómez D, Lozano M, Cubero J, Toribio-Delgado AF, Maynar-Mariño JI, Terrón MP, Muñoz JL, Pariente JA, Barriga C, Paredes SD, Rodríguez AB. A nutraceutical product based on Jerte Valley cherries improves sleep and augments the antioxidant status in humans. *Eur eJ Clin Nutr Metab* 4, e321-e323, 2009.

[74] Garrido M, Paredes SD, Cubero J, Lozano M, Toribio-Delgado AF, Muñoz JL, Reiter RJ, Barriga C, Rodríguez AB. Jerte valley cherry-enriched diets improve nocturnal rest and increase 6-sulfatoxymelatonin and total antioxidant capacity in the urine of middle-aged and elderly humans. *J Gerontol A: Biol Sci Med Sci* 65(9), 909-914, 2010.

[75] Maldonado MD, Moreno H, Calvo JR. Melatonin present in beer contributes to increase the levels of melatonin and antioxidant capacity of the human serum. *Clin Nutr* 28(2), 188-191, 2009.

[76] Tan DX, Manchester LC, Burkhardt S, Sainz RS, Mayo JC, Kohen R, Shohami E, Huo Y, Hardeland R, Reiter RJ. AFMK, a biogenic amine and melatonin metabolite, functions as a potent antioxidant. *FASEB J* 15(12), 2294-2296, 2001.

[77] Gitto E, Tan DX, Reiter RJ, Karbownik M, Manchester L, Cuzzocrea S, Fulia F, Barberi I. Individual and synergistic antioxidative actions of melatonin: studies with vitamin E, vitamin C, glutathione and desferoxamine in rat liver homogenates. *J Pharm Pharmacol* 53(10), 1393-1401, 2001.

[78] Galano A, Tan D, Reiter R. Melatonin as a natural ally against oxidative stress: a physicochemical examination. *J Pineal Res* 51(1), 1-16, 2011.

[79] Morreale M, Livrea MA. Synergistic effect of glycolic acid on the antioxidant activity of a-tocopherol and melatonin in lipid bilayers and in human skin homogenates. *Biochem Mol Biol Int* 42(6), 1093-1102, 1997.

[80] Blask DE, Sauer LA, Dauchy RT. Melatonin as a chronobiotic/ anticancer agent: cellular, biochemical and molecular mechanisms of action and their implications for circadian-based cancer therapy. *Curr Top Med Chem* 2(2), 113-132, 2002.

[81] Reiter RJ. Mechanisms of cancer inhibition by melatonin. *J Pineal Res* 37(3), 213-214, 2004.

[82] Kamdar BB, Tergas A, Mateen FJ, Bhayani NH, Oh J. Night-shift work and risk of breast cancer: a systematic review and meta-analysis. *Breast Cancer Res Treat* 138(1), 291-301, 2013.

[83] Rodríguez C, Martin V, Herrera F, García-Santos G, Rodríguez-Blanco J, Casado-Zapico S, Sanchez-Sanchez AM, Suárez S, Puente-Moncada N, Anítua M, Antolín I. Mechanisms involved in the pro-apoptotic effect of melatonin in cancer cells. *Int J Mol Sci* 14(4), 6597-6613, 2013.

[84] Anisimov V, Popovich I, Zabezhinski M, Anisimov S, Vesnushkin G, Vinogradova I. Melatonin as antioxidant, geroprotector and anticarcinogen. *Biochim Biophys Acta* 1757(5-6), 573-589, 2006.

[85] Pandi-Perumal SR, Trakht I, Srinivasan V, Spence DW, Maestroni GJM, Zisapel N, Cardinali DP. Physiological effects of melatonin: role of melatonin receptors and signal transduction pathways. *Progr Neurobiol* 85(3), 335-353, 2008.

[86] Miller SC, Pandi-Perumal SR, Esquifino AI, Cardinali DP, Maestroni GJM. The role of melatonin in inmmuno-enhancement: potential application in cancer. *Int J Exp Pathol* 87(2), 81-87, 2006.

[87] Jung-Hynes B, Reiter RJ, Ahmad N. Sirtuins, melatonin and circadian rhythms: building a bridge between aging and cancer. *J Pineal Res* 48(1), 9-19, 2010.

[88] Di Bella G, Mascia F, Gualano L, Di Bella L. Melatonin anticancer effects: Review. *Int J Mol Sci* 14, 2410-2430, 2013.

[89] Venegas C, García JA, Escames G, Ortiz F, López A, Doerrier C, García-Corzo L, López LC, Reiter RJ, Acuña-Castroviejo D. Extrapineal melatonin: analysis of its subcellular distribution and daily fluctuations. *J Pineal Res* 52(2), 217-227, 2012.

[90] Slominski A, Tobin DJ, Zmijewski MA, Wortsman J, Paus R. Melatonin in the skin: synthesis, metabolism and functions. *Trends Endocrinol Metabol* 19(1), 17-24, 2008.

[91] Tan DX, Manchester LC, Reiter RJ, Qi WB, Zhang M, Weintraub ST, Cabrera J, Saínz RM, Mayo JC. Identification of highly elevated levels of melatonin in bone marrow: its origin and significance. *Biochim Biophys Acta* 1472(1-2), 206-214, 1999.

[92] Raikhlin NT, Kvetnoy IM, Tolkachev VN. Melatonin may be synthesized in enterochromafinne cells. *Nature* 255(5506), 344-345, 1975.

[93] Konturek SJ, Konturek PC, Brzozowski T, Bubenik GA. Role of melatonin in upper gastrointestinal tract. *J Physiol Pharmacol* 58(Suppl 6), 23-52, 2007.
[94] Bubenik G. Gastrointestinal melatonin: localization, function, and clinical revelance. *Diges Dis Sci* 47(10), 2336-2348, 2002.
[95] Huether G. Melatonin synthesis in the gastrointestinal tract and the impact of nutritional factors on circulating melatonin. *Ann New York Acad Sci* 719, 146-158, 1994.
[96] Hardeland R, Pandi-Perumal SR. Melatonin, a potent agent in antioxidative defense: actions as a natural food constituent, gastrointestinal factor, drug and prodrug. *Nutr Metab* 2, 1-15, 2005.
[97] Oba S, Nakamura K, Sahashi Y, Hattori A, Nagata C. Consumption of vegetables alters morning urinary 6-sulfatoxymelatonin concentration. *J Pineal Res* 45(1), 17-23, 2008.
[98] Poeggeler B. Melatonin, aging, and age-related diseases: perspectives for prevention, intervention, and therapy. *Endocrine* 27(2), 201-212, 2005.
[99] Dahlitz M, Alvarez B, Vignau J, English J, Arendt J, Parkes J. Delayed sleep phase syndrome response to melatonin. *Lancet* 337(8750), 1121-1124, 1991.
[100] Dollins A, Zhdanova I, Wurtman R, Lynch H, Deng M. Effect of inducing nocturnal serum melatonin concentrations in daytime on sleep, mood, body temperature, and performance. *Proc Natl Acad Sci USA* 91(5), 1824-1828, 1994.
[101] Hardeland R, Madrid JA, Tan DX, Reiter RJ. Melatonin, the circadian multioscillator system and health: the need for detailed analysis of peripheral melatonin signal. *J Pineal Res* 52(2), 139-166, 2012.
[102] Takahashi T, Sasaki M, Itoh H, Ozone M, Yamadera W, Hayshida KI, Ushijima S, Matsunaga N, Obuchi K, Sano H. Effect of 3 mg melatonin on jet lag syndrome in an 8-h eastward flight. *Psychilatry Clin Neurosci* 54(3), 377-378, 2000.
[103] Herxheimer A. Jet lag. *Clin Evid* 13, 2178-2183, 2005.
[104] Bonnefont-Rousselot D, Collin F. Melatonin: Action as antioxidant and potential applications in human disease and aging. *Toxicology* 278(1), 55-67, 2010.
[105] Seabra M, Bignotto M, Pinto Jr L, Tufik S. Randomized double blind clinical trial, controlled with placebo, of the toxicology of chronic melatonin treatment. *J Pineal Res* 29(4), 193-200, 2000.

[106] Jan J, Hamilton D, Seward N, Fast D, Freeman R, Laudon M. Clinical trial of controlled-release melatonin in children with sleep-wake disorders. *J Pineal Res* 29(1), 34-39, 2000.

[107] Nordlund JJ, Lerner AB. The effects of oral melatonin on skin color and on the release of pituitary hormones. *J Clin Endocrinol Metab* 45(4), 768-774, 1977.

[108] Hugel HM, Kennaway DJ. Synthesis and chemistry of melatonin and of related compounds. A review. *Org Prep Proc Int* 27(1), 1-31, 1995.

[109] Prabhakar C, Vasanth-Kumar N, Ravikanth-Reddy M, Sarma RM, Om-Reddy G. Process research and development of melatonin. *Org Proc Res Dev* 3(3), 155-160, 1999.

[110] Thomson DW, Commeureuc AGJ, Berlin S, Murphy JA. Efficient route to the pineal hormone melatonin by radical-based indole synthesis. *Synth Commun* 33(20), 3631-3641, 2003.

[111] Williamson BL, Tomlinson AJ, Naylor S, Gleich GJ. Contaminats in commercial preparations of melatonin. *Mayo Clin Proc* 72(11), 1094-1095, 1997.

[112] Naylor S, Johnson KL, Williamson BL, Klarskov K, Gleich GJ. Structural characterization of contaminants in commercial preparations of melatonin by on-line HPLC-electrospray ionization-tandem mass spectrometry. *Adv Exp Med Biol* 467, 769-777, 1999.

[113] Williamson BL, Kenneth LJ, Tomlinson AJ, Gleich GJ, Naylor S. On-line HPLC-tandem mass spectrometry structural characterization of case associated contaminants of L-tryptophan implicated with the onset of eosinophilia-myalgia syndrome. *Toxicol Lett* 99(2), 139-150, 1988.

[114] Williamson BL, Tomlinson AJ, Mishra PK, Gleich GJ, Naylor S. Structural characterization of contaminants found in commercial preparations of melatonin: similarities to case-related compounds from L-tryptophan associated with Eosinophilia-Myalgia Syndrome. *Chem Res Toxicol* 11(3), 234-240, 1998.

[115] OECD-Organisation for Economic Co-operation & Development. Initial Assessment Report on Phthalimide. *Screening Information DataSet (SIDS)* SIAM 20, Paris, France, ID-85-41-6, 2006.

[116] Capello C, Fischer U, Hungerbühler K. What is a green solvent? A comprehensive framework for the environmental assesment of solvents. *Green Chem* 9, 927-934, 2007.

[117] Marioni F, Bertoli A, Pistelli L. A straightforward procedure to biosynthesise melatonin using freshly chopped *Achillea millefolium* L. as reagent. *Phytochem Lett* 1(2), 107-110, 2008.

EDITOR CONTACT INFORMATION

Noboru Motohashi, PhD
Former Professor and Director
Meiji Pharmaceutical University
Tokyo, Japan
Foreign Examiner
Evaluation of the PhD Thesis
Indian National University
India
Email: noborumotohashi@jcom.home.ne.jp

INDEX

B

D

E

F

G

H

I

J

K

L

M

N

O

P

S

T

U

V

W

X

Y

Z